Yanks, Shanks, and Mulligans

Golf Stories by a Country Doc

Jimmie Ashcraft, M.D.

Country Doctor Books
2437 Eastridge Drive
Billings, MT 59102

ISBN: 978-1-7345193-0-3

This book is printed on acid free paper.

Cover design and graphics by David Ashcraft

other books written by

Jimmie Ashcraft, M.D.

Reflections of a Country Doctor

The Next Prescription

Side Effects

Paging Dr. A

Dedicated to my grandchildren:

Garrett, Kendall, our angel Alexandra,
Rhianna, Owen, Isaac, and Ethan

and

to senior golfers everywhere

"As you walk down the fairway of life you must smell the roses, for you only get to play one round."

Ben Hogan

Contents

Preface

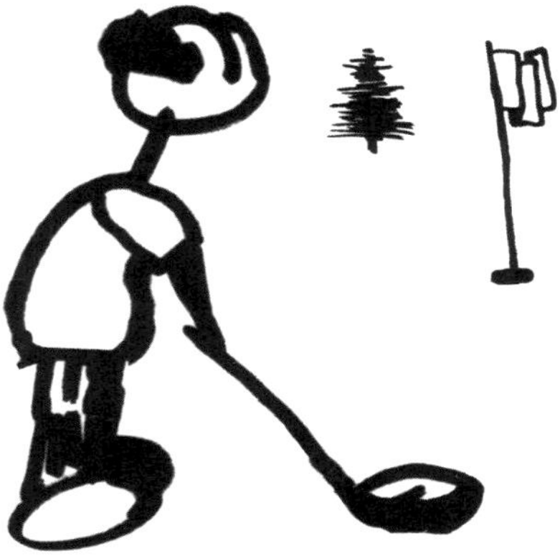

About six decades ago I was young man in Billings, Montana, taking a correspondence class to become an athletic trainer for the junior high school's athletic program. Physically, I was a runt. At 12 years of age I was barely 4 1/2 feet tall and weighed about 80 pounds. I definitely was not a student who was going to be a lineman on the football team or any player on the basketball team. However, I was smart. I wanted to be the guy who fixed my classmates when they got injured. Also, my mother knew I couldn't get hurt being an athletic trainer. This course was my inspiration to be a physician. The direction of my life was set.

In a blink of an eye, I fast forward through college, getting married, medical school, helping to raise three children, working decades as a country doctor in a rural Montana community and a lifelong educator, to my current situation of an energetic senior citizen entering the eighth decade of his life. Who would have guessed that my brothers and I would have lived this long if they only understood the circumstances under which we grew up? If we couldn't play with a bat and ball or just a ball, then we didn't play. Playing golf was never on my radar. Anyway, my brothers and I survived and prospered.

What do I do with myself now that I'm retired from caring for people in my medical practice? My younger brother encouraged me to take up golf because it was the second hardest thing I would ever do. Besides coping with aging and the bodily changes that accompany it, I have to admit that golf is a pretty tough second. Aging and golf are definitely not for pantywaists.

Previously, I wrote four books with collections of true stories about my experiences from my medical practice. One day in the fall of 2019 I had an inspiration to write a book about my experiences while golfing just for fun.

I certainly was not the best senior golfer around since I had been playing consistently only since I retired, a mere few years. Some of the men with whom I had played golf had been involved with the game since they were six years old; they were doggone good! Some of these fellows had captured club championships, senior club championships, and even statewide golf championships. I learned that these players were incredible silent mentors of the game of golf if I just sat back, kept quiet, watched, and listened to everything they did while they played. In fact, I discovered that if I really paid attention, I learned an awful lot from every golfer.

Additionally, I witnessed and heard a considerable amount about the human experience every time I played golf with someone. Every person I ever played with had a story. The golf course proved to be a wonderful place to learn about these stories. I have collected some of these accounts and put them into this book. Some golfer's narratives were just too personal to write about, so I omitted them. However, I want all these individuals to know that I appreciate their confidence in me by relating their very personal stories.

This book is a collection of stories and events that I witnessed while golfing.

My son David made the original graphics and cover for the book after my instructions to "make the book fun." I think he accomplished just what his old Dad had in mind.

Although the text was reviewed by others, including my best friend and amazing wife Kay whose input was superb as usual, I assume sole responsibility for the final content.

"One of the most fascinating things about golf is how it reflects the cycle of life. No matter what you shoot - the next day you have to go back to the first tee and begin all over again and make yourself into something."
Peter Jacobsen

Introduction

The hardest game any of us will ever play is the game of life. When we are young we don't give much thought to the game of life and its predetermined outcome. As a physician I cared for many who tried to prevent, prolong, destroy, or deny life's inevitable results with whatever potion, exercise, medication, religion, treatment, or whatever they could find. The natural behavior for self-preservation is powerful, but sometimes it can lead to unfortunate situations. I understood, however, that no matter what my patients did to slow down Mother Time, the end result of the game of life was the always same.

I was born in 1948. At that time, the average life expectancy for men in America was about 60 years, if everything worked out perfectly. As I write this book, I have survived a decade beyond my life expectancy of 1948 by shear good luck I guess.

Not too long ago I visited a young female physician who told me I looked young for my age. I thanked the woman for her kind words and told her I really should be dead at my age. I related I was well past my life expectancy when I was born, and, statistically, I should be dead. I mentioned that I was in the fourth quarter of my life's game, and, who knew, I could be in sudden-death overtime.

The doctor was taken aback by my comments apparently because she had never thought of her patients in that way and since she cared for mostly elderly people. She told me that I obviously wasn't dead yet, so we would just have to deal with what I had left. We both laughed.

Soon after I retired from my active medical practice, my brother John, who had been playing golf since his college days and was an assistant at a golf school in Arizona, forcefully encouraged me to find something else to do with my time; he knew I just would not and could not remain dormant. He suggested that I come to Arizona for a week to take some golf lessons and "learn to play the most difficult game I would ever know."

Being contrary, I told him that the game of life was the most difficult game that I knew of because that's what I had been doing for the last 40 years of my life in medicine.

John agreed. He continued to tell me that I would find golf to be the "second most difficult game in my life." (I should mention now that my brother John is a reasonably accomplished golfer. At the time of the writing of this book, he remains a low handicap player, has won multiple golf club championships, and has nine holes-in-one to his credit.) I, like most golfers, am still hoping to experience my first hole-in-one moment.

During my medical practice years I was too busy to play golf regularly. Kay and I would usually play for fun only a few times a year at charity events or while we were away vacationing. I have to admit that most of the time we were taking pictures of the scenery, the people, and flowers and not putting much real effort into the golf games.

I took the bait and attended a John Jacobs golf school in Green Valley, Arizona. When the school started, the PGA professional teaching the class took videos of his students. While we were viewing the initial video of my swinging a driver, the instructor said, "You played a lot of baseball didn't you?"

When I told him I had played baseball for as long as I could remember, he said, "It will take a lot of practice on your part, but I think we can fix your swing."

I have to admit that the golf lessons were difficult. I am an academic analytic thinker who evaluates just about everything. The golf pro kept telling me to be loosen up, be natural, and "let your body just do its thing."

I had to tell him that there was actually nothing natural about the golf swing; my body was doing its thing!

He had to agree with me on that point.

Each day after class, my brother took me out to play golf on the course for the remainder of the day until sunset. He made sure that I practiced what I have been taught during the day's lessons. We then went to the clubhouse restaurant to have a debriefing for the day. I had a soda, and he had a beer. (I figured he needed a beer or two after putting up with my yanks, shanks, cuts, flops, divots, sky balls, and mulligans for the entire day.)

On the last day of the lessons, the golf pro emphasized that we would not be very good for a while. In fact, he said we would probably be a lot worse than when we started. This statement did not impress me a bit. I wondered, "How could I get worse?"

Boy was he right! I spent so much time thinking about stance, alignment, the terrain, the wind, and anything else I could factor into my golf equation that I forgot to just hit the ball the best that I could. It took me a while to improve. A long while.

The following spring I reread the golf manual from my golf class. I practiced my golf swing in my garage until the Montana winter's snow melted. Then I went outside on my lawn to practice more. I went to the driving range a few times at the nearby golf club to practice, but I found this process tedious, boring, and emotionally unsatisfactory. Consequently, I purchased a year's playing membership at the golf club. I found that playing golf by myself on the course was a much better way for me to practice and to concentrate on what I had been taught. Playing alone was also a wonderful way for me to enjoy the beauty and wonders of nature. (Before attending medical school, I was a biologist.)

Somewhere along the way, I met some senior golfers who really didn't care how badly I played. They just joked when I hit a big banana slice into a lake; or when I hit the big ball (the earth) before I hit the little ball thus producing a gigantic hole in the ground called a divot or, in my case, a crater! Even if I had a lucky drive that went straight down the fairway 300 yards. (Yes, I did hit a few 300 yard drives with my persimmon 1-wood when I was younger and more flexible. Some of the shots even landed on the fairway.) The guys just wanted me to loosen up and enjoy myself playing golf.

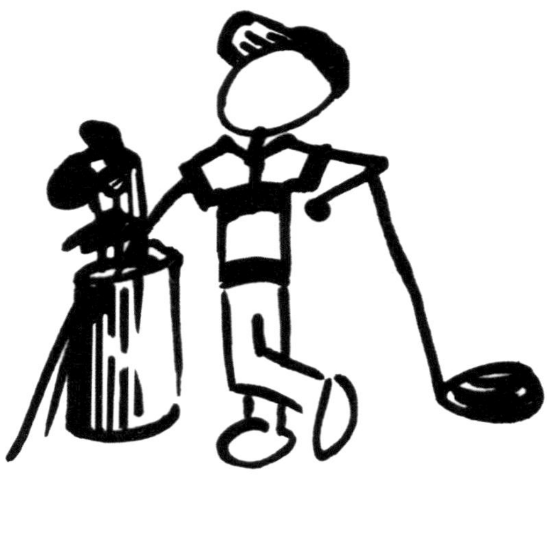

Soon, my golf game improved a little. More important to me, however, were the personal aspects of the players I had the pleasure to meet. While playing, I heard stories of personal and family tragedies that changed the lives of my playing companions. I perceived that golf became a temporary reprieve and sanctuary from their many worries. I appreciated the courage of the human spirit from these individuals that was far more important to me, as a person and a physician, than my learning how to play golf better. Furthermore, I witnessed some goofy events and many golfer shenanigans that brightened my days. Along the way, somehow, my golf scores and performance improved dramatically.

I never played golf a single day without learning something new about nature, the game of golf, or about the people I was privileged to meet. At the end of each golf match, I still thank each of the players for "the lessons."

This book contains a few stories about my experiences while playing senior golf as an old doc. I have changed the names of the individuals in the stories for confidentiality. I certainly have no intention of embarrassing anybody except me. However, all the episodes in the book did occur.

ENJOY!

"Golf is deceptively simple and endlessly complicated;
it satisfies the soul and frustrates the intellect.
It is at the same time rewarding and maddening
– and it is without a doubt the greatest
game mankind has ever invented."
Arnold Palmer

A Wee Bit of History

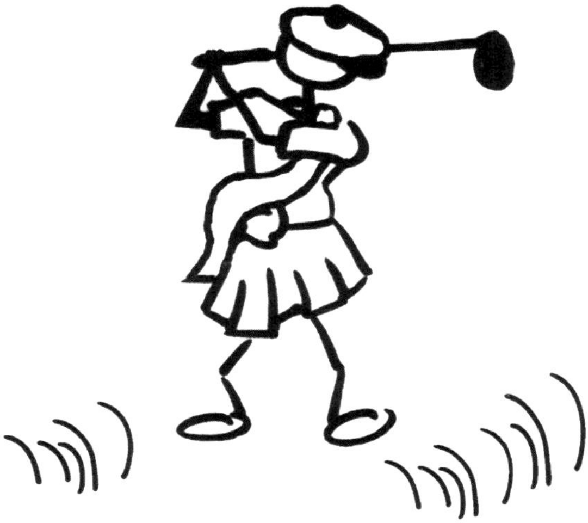

Sometime during the 1600s Scottish shepherds must have become bored as they moved their flocks from one field to the next, so they started to hit stones and whatever else was in their way with sticks. Eventually, being the competitive bunch that they were, the Scots decided to make their stone hitting exercise into a game.

The very first recorded golf tournament played under a written set of rules was at Leith Links in Scotland near present-day Edinburgh in 1744. The course had five holes and was played twice or thrice. Those rules included these pearls:

"If a ball be stopped by any person, horse, dog, or anything else, the ball so stopped must be played where it lies."

"Neither Trench, Ditch or Dyke, made for the preservation of the Links, nor the Scholar's Holes, or the Soldier's Lines, ShAll be accounted a Hazard; But the ball is to be taken out, teed and play'd with any Iron Club."

The Ancient Golf Club at St. Andrews in Scotland is considered the home of modern-day golf. It was founded by 22 Scottish gentlemen in 1754. In 1834, King William IV of England conferred his patronage upon the club and it became the Royal and Ancient Golf Club (R&A). In 1897 the first rules of golf committee was established and the R&A became the official recognized governing body for golf throughout the world except in the United States. Today the R&A works together with United States Golf Association (USGA) to set the standards and rules of the game around the world.

"The proper score for a businessman golfer is 90. If he is better than that he is neglecting his business. If he's worse, he's neglecting his golf."

-St Andrews Rotary Club Member

The Game

Going from playing baseball and softball for most of my life to playing golf was a physical, mental, and cultural shock. Not only did I have to learn a new set of rules but I had to learn to swing a stick attached to a club head in the most unorthodox manner. I had to learn and communicate with a new language. Additionally, I needed to learn, to walk, to dress, to talk, to sneeze, and to stand up straight at the appropriate times, places, and meters.

For example, when your golfing partner hits a ball that curves severely to the right and into a lake after hitting a tree, another golfer in your group who is fixated on the rulebook could say something like, "Goodness, Henry, it appears that your ball in play, struck from the teeing ground with your 1-wood, has crossed the margin of the water hazard after hitting that tree, designated by the red wooden stakes and line. According to official rule # 4.XYZ.6, this entitles you to five relief options, one of which is to measure two club lengths from the spot the ball entered the water and drop it there. You will be assessed a one stroke penalty." This verbiage may be totally correct. I have played with golfers who, I was convinced, had the golf rule book memorized, carried it at all times, and talked just like this whenever a ruling was needed.

However, in time I learned by watching more seasoned golfers respond to rule interpretations that, to not appear like a total idiot in front of his playing companions, one player might say, "Henry, you shanked your shot into a tree and it fell into the lake. Just drop a ball where it went in and take your one stroke penalty." Certainly, this comment is far less refined, but totally accurate, more easily understood, and equally acceptable for the situation. Easy answers also speed up the pace of play. In time, I believe each golfer develops his or her own unique golf language.

I learned that the average recreational golfer shoots a score of approximately 100 or more. Also, while learning how to swing my golf club to the cadence of saying, "John-ny Mil-ler, John-ny Mil-ler," I calculated that it takes only about two-seconds per golf swing. That means, it only takes about 200 seconds, or about 3 1/2 minutes, to perform all the hitting to be done during an 18-hole golf round. When the typical golf match lasts about four hours, what the heck fills in the rest of the time? In time, I found out that the remainder of the time is used up with warming up, talking, joking, searching for golf balls, walking, riding in a golf cart, keeping score, relaxing, having something to eat and drink, gambling, going to the bathroom, enjoying the views of nature that the golf course provides, thinking, and most importantly interacting with your fellow golfers. I came to appreciate that golf is a game of unwritten rules and outdated stereotypes, and becoming familiar with all that "stuff" was a challenging task at best. I found out that to be comfortable at the golf course, I had to become proficient at and be committed to the entire process.

There were so many common golf terms that had other real world meanings. As a novice, I had to learn about winter rules, what was an apron in golf, what were cuts, yips, yanks, shanks, slices, chips, flops, mulligans, and hazards just to name a few new golf terms. Soon, my score became my secondary concern.

I discovered that the game of golf is not just hitting the ball and counting up the number of times you hit it. It encompasses a vast array of games with names like 2-best-balls, 3-best-balls, scramble, shamble, red-white-blue, waltz time, stroke play, match play, Stableford, and many more. To complicate matters, each of these games has multiple local club *modifications* to the basic rules.

Ah, yes, and the bewildering task of trying to choose the "best" golf ball. They are all round with dimples in various patterns. They all are the same weight and size. But what color do I choose? What about a harder ball or a softer one? What is golf ball spin rate anyway? Is it important to me, and, if so, how do I control it? I just can't begin to discuss all the kinds and variations of golf clubs, the irons, woods, and hybrids, because they seem to change EVERY YEAR!

Years ago, a good friend named Earl Neff who had played golf from the age of four until he was almost ninety told me, "Jim, golf was made to be a game for gentlemen. So darn it, act like one!" In Earl's memory I try.

*"If you're not confused,
you're not paying attention."*
Tom Peters

The Golf Landscape

Golf is indeed a confusing game. Very little comes naturally or instinctively. Every golf course is a nature preserve with natural and man-made components. Each course has a collection of groomed areas called holes that are given a number. Every numbered hole on the golf course (usually 9 or 18) has another hole dug into a groomed and flattened grassy surface called the green. This hole supports a flag-bearing pole called a flagstick that gets moved on a daily basis, sometimes.

A ball that is hit "*through the green*" can actually still be on the green. Every hole on the golf course has a handicap score and every player has a course handicap that varies according to the golf course. A lateral water hazard does not necessarily have water in it. A bunker is not a place to hide during an air raid, but is a dugout spot in the ground that may be filled with grass or sand. These areas ARE NOT to be called 'traps.'

No two golf courses are the same. In fact, I would guess that no two golf courses are even similar. Besides, each golf course changes on a daily basis depending upon the temperature, the wind velocity and its direction, the air humidity, the number of leaves or animals on the ground, and innumerable other environmental factors. Therefore, a similar golf shot on the same hole from an identical place may be totally different from one day to the next or even from one hour to the next depending upon the circumstances.

Over the years I developed innate muscle memories for striking a round ball with my wooden bat playing baseball and softball. I found that old muscle memories are hard to modify when I started trying to swing a golf club. My body and mind told me that hitting down on the ball would make the ball go down and hitting up on the ball would produce a fly ball. In golf, however, the mechanism is just the opposite. Hitting down on the ball makes it go up into the air and hitting up on the ball frequently makes the ball curve downward into the ground.

Is my body confused yet? Absolutely!

Over time I heard the various names of the different golf clubs. The Driver or 1-wood (which is actually made of metal now) is also referred to as "the Big Dog," "Old Numero Uno," "the big boy," "the fat boy," "the showtime stick," and others. The putter can be called "the flat stick," "the old equalizer," "the money maker," and "the magic wand."

Furthermore, the game of golf has many redundant terms. A "slice," or a right deviation of a mishit shot from a right-handed golfer, is not a piece of pie. In golf a 'slice' is also called a cut, a banana ball, a chop, a block, a fade, a shank, a fan, a push, a curve, a slash, and perhaps more.

To make matters more confusing to me, to make the ball go farther the golfer uses a club with a lower number. To hit the ball a shorter distance a club with a higher number is used. When a golfer "clubs up" he actually chooses a golf club with a lower number, and when he chooses to "club down" he reaches for a club with a higher number. In baseball, the harder one swings his bat and hits the ball, the ball usually goes farther. In golf, however, swinging the club with less force frequently makes the golf ball go farther.

Finally, the day comes when you have a breakthrough. You firmly believe that you have mastered a golf swing that is repeatable with somewhat predictable scoring. In the middle of a round the Montana spring weather changes! The gentle breeze changes direction and intensifies to a tropical force gale. Tree pollen plugs up your nose. Your eyes start to have tears from the flying dirt. The temperature drops 20°. Your arthritis flares. The aching from an old back injury decides to resurface. You accidentally step into a hole on the course and twist an ankle or knee. You try a little harder against the wind and those doggone long-lost muscle memories of your baseball days return with a vengeance. The forgotten, or should I say misplaced, yanks and shanks are reborn! You finally realize that all of a sudden you have trouble putting both of your hands in your back pockets at the same time. Such is golf.

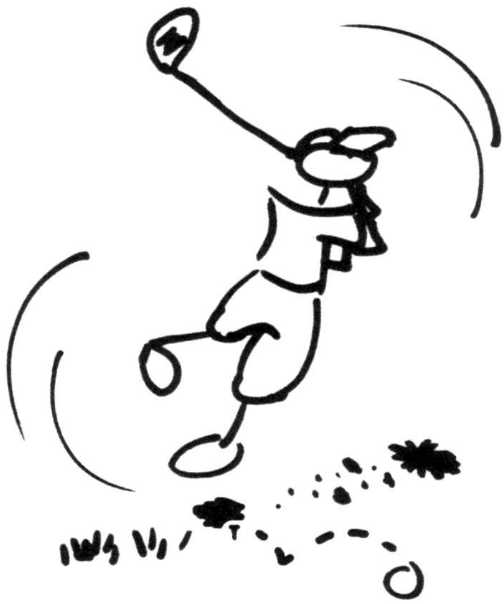

"Reverse every natural instinct and do the opposite of what you are inclined to do, and you will probably come very close to having a perfect golf swing."

Ben Hogan

My First Golf Game

I was a 24-year-old sophomore in medical school the first time I played golf. One of my classmates named Larry asked me to play a round of golf with him one day because he said no one else wanted to oblige him. I told him that I had never played golf and that I did not have a set of clubs. Actually, I really knew nothing about the game of golf except one hits a ball into a hole with a club. I was also a destitute medical student, *and I emphasize poor*, because my wife Kay and I literally had no money to spend for extra activities let alone playing golf.

Larry assured me that it was going to cost me only $5. I could also rent clubs at the golf course if I needed. Larry begged me to play with him because he repeated that no one else would play with him. He gave a convincing speech, but I knew full well that I had no idea how to play the game, and I did not have a set of golf clubs. I told him I would let him know the next day.

I discussed the request with my wife Kay who was pregnant at the time with our first child. She told me we could make the budget work and gave me her blessing to play. Apparently, Kay thought I needed a break from the rigors of my medical school studies. I called Larry and told him that I could play golf with him. He arranged a tee time at a nearby golf course for the coming weekend when we were both off duty for any medical school commitments.

I had no golf clubs, but Peter, a neighbor in our apartment complex, had a set of clubs that I had noticed in his storage cage that was in the basement of our condominium units. I explained to Peter my situation, and he readily offered to let me use his golf clubs for the day. He even offered to let me use the balls that were in the golf bag. Additionally, he gave me a written note telling me how far he could hit the ball with each golf club. Finally, Peter gave me a few basic tips on swinging the golf club.

Larry and I traveled to the golf course together. Upon our arrival, he gave me the basic layout of the course and explained to me some of the rudimentary rules for playing. After a short warm-up at the practice range, we headed to the first tee box.

Larry gave me the "honor" of playing first. He informed me that the player who had the lowest score on the current hole received the *honor* for the next hole. I guess he figured that he would have the honor for each hole after the initial tee off since I had never played the game.

Looking down a wide open fairway banked on both sides by trees, as I recall, I used the driver for my first ever golf shot. Remembering my days hitting baseballs, I kept my head still, concentrated on the golf ball and swung the golf club hard hoping for the best. Amazingly, the ball traveled down the left side of the fairway and faded to the right a bit before landing toward the middle of the fairway.

Larry asked, "Are you sure you never played golf before?"

I swore that I had never played before.

Larry got up to the first tee box with his driver and made a mighty left-handed swing. I was standing just opposite and behind him a bit when he hit the ball. His golf ball went straight sideways hitting me in the right leg and ricocheted out of bounds.

Larry said, "Oops."

He repeated his tee shot which barely traveled beyond the ladies' tee box. (I would learn later that he should have taken a penalty stroke for hitting his first golf ball out-of-bounds.)

On the first par 4 hole I had a bogey 5. I thought to myself, "Not too bad for a fella who had never hit a golf ball before." Larry's problems hitting the ball continued, and he scored an 8.

Two holes later I stood behind Larry's back to make sure I would not get hit again. Amazingly, when he hit the ball, it went sideways between his legs and hit me in the left leg! I was beginning to understand why people did not want to play with Larry. It was downright dangerous.

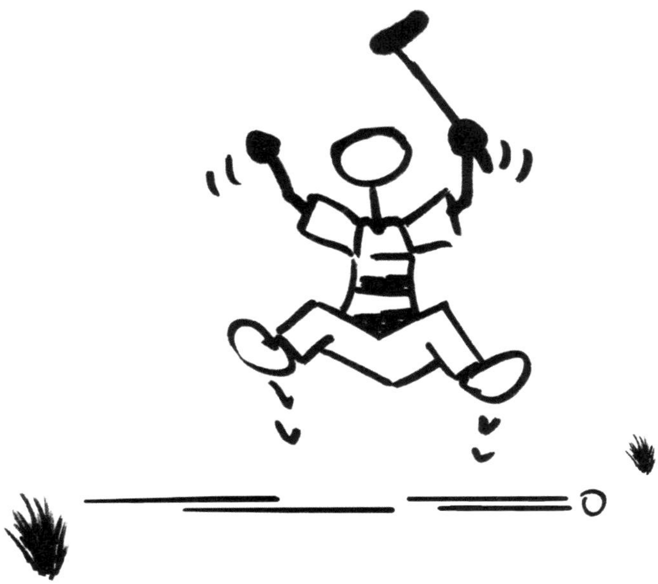

As I recall, my very best shot was when I hit a long drive that rolled a bit and settled a short distance off the fairway a few feet from a tree. I hit my ball solidly with a 3-wood. The ball screamed out of the rough and landed just in front of the green before it rolled about 3 feet away from the flagstick. I hit the ball in for a birdie 4 on a par five. Larry took a 10 on this hole.

As we worked our way through the remainder of the golf of course, Larry continued to struggle mightily while I was pleasantly surprised at how well I could strike the golf ball. My final score for the first time I ever played golf was 84, twelve strokes over par. Larry, however, scored his apparent usual at 114. Larry was convinced that I had lied to him and I was a real sandbagger (someone who claims to be worse than he really is to gain strokes). What could I say? He was uncoordinated and couldn't play well.

Anyway, I played with Larry once more a couple weeks later with similar results. It would be the last I would play golf until I finished medical school and my internship year, and I was serving in the National Health Service Corps in the wilds of Wyoming.

I Used to Play Pretty Fair

It was the early spring. I had completed my one-week instructional golf school in Green Valley, Arizona with my brother the fall before; I was eager to work on all the things I had been taught. I called the golf course to find a time that was not very busy so I could take my time practicing and playing. I arrived at the golf course with ample time to loosen up before my tee time.

The golf pro tending the counter at the golf shop that morning asked me if I would be willing to play with an older gentleman.

I informed him that I just wanted to practice on things I had learned at the golf school. I was not very good; I was not prepared to play with a partner.

The golf pro assured me that the fellow I would be playing with would not mind a bit. In fact, he probably would enjoy my company.

I agreed and off to first tee box I walked.

I met a diminutive gentleman on the first tee box I guessed to be almost 80 years old. I was just 60 years old at the time. The golfer told me his name was Marcus Sullivan, and he appreciated having a companion while he played.

Mr. Sullivan went to the tee box, took out his 1-wood, and blasted his golf ball down the middle of the fairway about 200 yards. I thought to myself, "This old guy looks like he's pretty good." I then got up to the tee box, took a mighty swing, and laced my ball about 270 yards downrange. Unfortunately, the shot had a considerable slice, and I ended up about 30° off-line in the heavy grass on the right side of the fairway.

As we marched down the fairway together toward our respective golf balls, Marcus asked me what I did for a living. I informed him that I had practiced medicine in rural Sidney, Montana, for a quarter-century and then served as a medical educator for another five years. I had retired after putting in 80 to 100-hour weeks for almost 45 years. I mentioned that I had taken a course to learn how to play golf the fall before. I hoped he didn't mind my practicing the things I had been taught in the golf school.

Marcus told me I could practice all I wanted while we played. Then he wanted to know if I was a "real medical doctor."

I told him that yes, I had practiced real country doctor medicine. I made home visits out in the country. I assisted mothers giving birth. I performed major surgery. I cared for high-risk newborn infants and intensive care cardiac patients. I straightened fractured arms and legs. I performed many other duties that needed to be done in a rural Montana town.

Mr. Sullivan told me that he was glad to be playing with me. He said he would tell me part of his story after we finished the first hole. We then walked to our respective golf balls. He was in the middle of the fairway. My ball landed far to the right of the fairway in the middle of some 4-inch-deep grass.

Marcus hit his second shot quite low and the ball ran up to the edge of the green. I hacked away at my shot in the rough and somehow the golf gods decided it should land on the green.

Marcus chipped his ball to within a foot or so of the flagstick, and then tapped his ball in for par. Using my very best putting technique I learned in golf school, I three putted for a bogey.

We then made our way to the second tee box. En route, Mr. Sullivan told me that he worked in marketing for many years. He had played golf since he was a small boy. He remarked, "I used to play pretty fair." Marcus then said, sort of as an aside, "A few medical issues along the way slowed me down a bit."

We teed off again. Marcus was again in the middle of the fairway, and I was somewhere in the trees to the right of the fairway. As we walked together down the fairway, Marcus started to relate his medical history in brief. Apparently, one day while golfing ten years before he collapsed on the golf course and had to be resuscitated. He had suffered a heart attack. Marcus maintained that he woke up in the hospital after two stents had been inserted into his heart arteries. About five years after this episode, Marcus told me he felt sort of funny one day and went to see his family doctor. The doctor thought he had an upset stomach and sent him home with some medicines. Reassured that all was good, Marcus proceeded to mow his lawn. He told me that he collapsed in the middle of his front yard, was found by a neighbor, and woke up after a triple bypass operation. He had no recollection of any the events.

Marcus thought that if someone was having a heart attack, the person would experience some sort of pain. He told me he had no discomfort whatsoever.

I informed him that only about 20% of people having heart attacks report having chest discomfort. Additionally, about 20% of people with acute heart attacks have no discomfort whatsoever.

Marcus confided to me that no one had ever told him that. He thought, maybe, he should not have fired his family doctor for not making the correct diagnosis.

I just listened to his story as we walked.

For his second shot, Marcus hit the ball again quite low and it again rolled onto the green. Unfortunately, the green was large and his ball was a long way from the flagstick which was located at the back edge of the green.

After hitting a shot, Marcus came up to me to see my situation in the trees. My ball was lying about 100 yards from the flagstick, but trees were a few yards in front of me. He asked me what I was planning to do for my next shot. I really had no idea. I considered hitting the ball sideways onto the fairway, or just blasting away to see if I could launch the ball over the trees. He then suggested that I choke up on my 5 iron, place the ball near my back foot and hit down on the ball so that it would *scoot* under all the trees. I gave it a try, and it worked! My ball landed in the middle of the green.

Despite the long distance for his putt, Marcus managed a par. I too made a two-putt par. We congratulated each other. I thanked Marcus for the golfing tip.

As we walked toward the next tee box, Marcus told me that he was physically able to play only nine holes of golf at a time since his stroke three years before. He apparently had a paralysis of his left side that mostly resolved with time and physical therapy. He also had surgeries on the arteries in his neck to improve blood flow to his head. To make his point, Marcus showed me the scars on both sides of his neck.

I was starting to think this guy might collapse on me at any time. I asked myself, "Was that why the golf pro wanted me to play with him?"

The third hole was a 160-yard par 3. Marcus bounced his golf ball close to the flagstick which was placed near the front of the green. I was on the far side of the green and a long way from the flagstick. Marcus executed a nice curving putt for a birdie! I made three outstanding putts for a bogey!

The fourth hole was a 500-yard par five. Both of our drives ended up in the middle of the fairway. For Marcus this was the usual event. For me, it appeared to be a gift from the golf gods. As we walked toward our golf balls in the middle of the fairway, Marcus told me that another reason he could play only nine holes was because he had to get home to care for his wife who recently suffered a stroke. He was able to golf only during her morning nap which usually lasted about three hours. He said a neighbor watched her while he was away just in case something happened. We both had a par five on this hole.

As we walked toward the #5 hole Marcus said, "Jim, it's obvious to me from looking at your golf swing that you used to play baseball. Do not worry. It will take time, but your golf swing will improve. When you practice remember that quality is always better than quantity. Give yourself plenty of time and just be patient."

Marcus scored a par 3 on this hole. I shot a double bogey 5. I blamed the slope of the green.

As we played the remaining holes I could see that Marcus was getting tired. The weakness in his left arm and leg became more prevalent, but he did not complain. As we finished the final hole and shook hands, Marcus apologized for not playing as well the last few holes. I could see that his decline in performance bothered him significantly.

Marcus finished the nine holes with a score of 3 over par. I was 8 over par. I thought to myself, "This guy is almost 20 years older than me, he has suffered two heart attacks and a stroke, AND today he beat me easily by 5 strokes."

As we were walking off the green toward the clubhouse, Marcus repeated, "I used to play pretty fair.

I'm just lucky to be here, I guess. Thank you for playing with me, and listening to an old man ramble on."

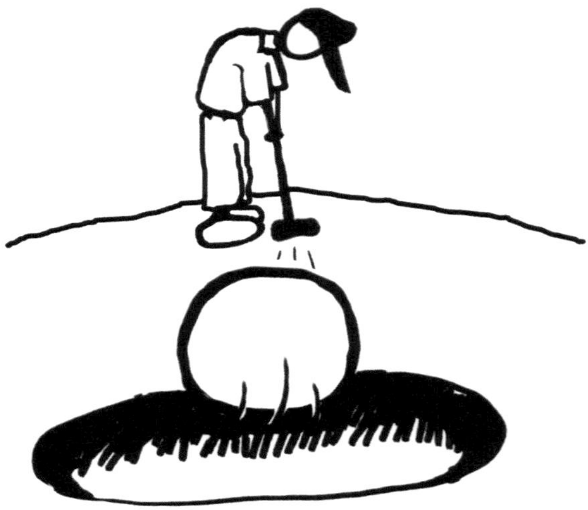

I replied to Mr. Sullivan, "Thank you for the lessons." I'm sure he thought I meant the golf lessons. I assumed he had no idea that I was evaluating him from my medical perspective the entire time we were playing. He taught me a lot about golf and the resilience of one man this day.

From this day forward I have continued to thank people at the end of each golf round for "the lessons." I am sure they are thinking only about golf lessons. However, I can never tell my fellow golfers how much I learn from them about the human spirit and the game of golf each and every time I play.

"Golf is a game that's played on a 5 inch course—the distance between your ears."
Bobby Jones

The First Foursome

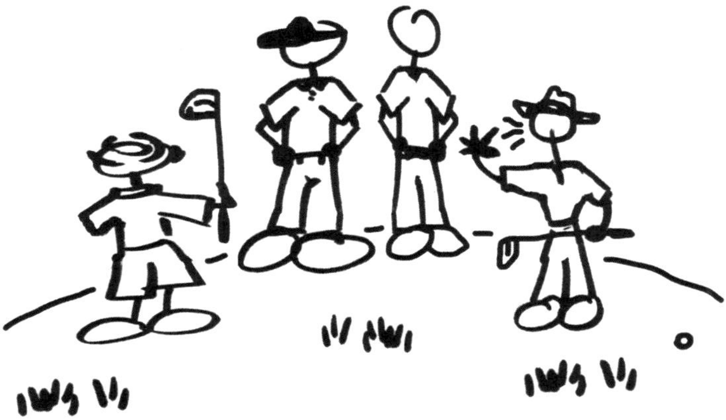

Earl and Mike joined me on the 10th hole on a gorgeous spring day in May. There was no wind, there were a few clouds, and all I wanted to do was practice the drills I had learned at a golf school in Arizona the previous fall. These two golfers had already played the first nine holes of the course; I was planning to play just the second nine holes. As soon as they arrived at the tee box and introduced themselves, Earl started to recruit me to play in the senior golf league. I informed him that I was just learning how to play golf and that I really wasn't into the competitive nature of sports.

Both men, especially Earl, emphasized that the senior golf league was nothing like the cutthroat men's league which played at a different time of day. The senior league, which included only players over the age of 55 years and mostly retired, always played in the mornings when most people were working. This pair emphasized vigorously that the senior league always wanted new old players.

I didn't give them much encouragement that I would become involved. However, my indifferent attitude did not dissuade these two gentlemen. Earl and Mike made fun of me, my golf shots, and themselves, in a good-natured way, for the next two hours.

Mike was hunched over. I could see he had a stiff neck and a hand tremor. Mike said the orthopedic surgeons fixed his neck to be stiff so he could keep his eye on the golf ball. He quipped that he used to be 6 feet 2 inches tall before seven back surgeries made him 5 feet 6 inches. Apparently, he had multiple other medical issues also, but outwardly he was always telling jokes and played the best he could. He said he used to have dreams of how his life would be, but his GOD had a different plan for him.

Earl was a thin fellow in his sixties I guessed. He continually made fun of himself, Mike, and me in between puffs on a cigarette. Earl played quite well this day as I recall. This duo was determined to disrupt my concentration on playing golf this day, and they succeeded magnificently. I did not hit the ball well. However, I did have a fun time playing with them.

When we were finished, Earl told me when and where I could sign-up for the senior golf league.

I made no commitments.

I discussed my encounter on the golf course with these guys with my wife Kay. She thought it might be good for me to at least check out the senior golf league if for no other reason than to get me out of the house and socialize a bit. I had always been a non-social animal, a nerd if you will, who was content to take care of his patients, his medical practice, and his family. I decided to take the plunge and sign up for senior golf. I figured the worst I would have to do was quit. Quitting, however, had never been in my vocabulary. My wife and I both knew that if I got into something I would do it with 100% of my energy.

I contacted Earl with the phone number he had provided and advised him that I was willing to participate in the senior league just to see what would happen. Earl told me to show up the next Monday morning. He said tee time was at 8 am, so I should come early enough to have time to register, pay my fees, and warm-up. The cost to play every Monday morning was the princely sum of four dollars. For an additional dollar I could participate in the 'deuce pot' lottery. In addition, I would have to pay green fees for the day or purchase a yearly pass to the golf club.

I appeared at 7 am the next Monday morning at the golf course. I was directed to the attendant at the club shop to pay the appropriate fees. Afterward, the nice lady directed me downstairs to sign in for the day's senior league event. Earl was sitting at the table and, when I appeared, he produced a big cheesy grin on his face. He said, "You told me you weren't into playing in a highly competitive environment. After your round today, I want you to tell me how it was." Earl said my group started on the 3rd tee box which was as far west from the clubhouse as I could walk and still be on the golf course. Then he pointed his arm due west and told me to start walking. Earl let me know that the other three players would be riding carts.

My three playing companions were already on the tee box waiting for me when I arrived. I met Barney first. He was a gentleman about 75 years old; he was almost blind. He asked me if I would consider driving his cart because of his poor vision.

I agreed.

Barney pointed out the other members of our foursome. He told me that Delbert, who was almost 80, was quite deaf even with his hearing aids in place. Therefore, when I talked to Delbert, I was instructed to first get his attention and then look him straight in the eyes so he could read my lips.

The other member of the foursome was Albert. Barney said that there was nothing physically wrong with Albert, but he had serious memory issues. After I got his attention and spoke to him directly, Delbert repeated that Albert appeared absolutely normal but his attention span was zilch. Delbert told me that he and Albert had been friends forever. Apparently, Delbert always drove Albert in the golf cart when they played together because his friend was easily confused.

The activities of the blind fellow and the deaf fellow were reasonably managed while we played. However, Albert caused our group a considerable amount of difficulty. He would hit a ball but could not remember where it went. When he was left unattended in the golf cart Albert would take off across the golf course and pick up any golf ball he found, including those of his playing partners. We had to determine who the balls belonged to and where to replace them. To say the least, this erratic activity caused our foursome to spend a lot of extra time on the golf course in places we should never have been. In fact, when we finally arrived back in the clubhouse, we were almost 1/4 hour behind the last group to check-in.

Earl was waiting for me at the event table. He asked me how our round went. Looking at our scorecard Earl laughed and declared, "I see you guys scored, not well, but you did have a score."

Trying not to laugh, I tried to recreate for Earl our foursome's golf adventure for the day.

He then asked, "Jim, now wasn't that about the most competitive round of golf you ever had?" Again, he produced a big cheesy smile and laughed out loud.

To be sure, our team did not win any prizes that day. In fact, we were about 10 strokes worse than the lowest score recorded.

Afterward, I had to admit that I did have a good time. I decided to continue playing senior league golf.

"You don't have the game you played last year or last week. You only have today's game. It may be far from your best, but that's all you've got. Harden your heart and make the best of it."

Walter Hagen

Integrity

Our foursome was about ready to tee off on our ninth and last hole of the morning. Jackson, one of the members of our foursome, was having a marvelous scoring outing. His usual senior league handicap was about 8 which meant his usual score was about 8 strokes over par for nine holes. Today, Jackson walked to the ninth tee box with a running score of one over par. All he had to do on the ninth hole to beat his very best ever score was to get a bogey 5.

The ninth hole on the second nine is about 370 yards long with a slight dog leg turn to the left. If a tee shot strays too far to the right it ventures into either a lake or knee-deep grass. If the ball is hit too far to the left it goes into an area with trees, hills, and some deep grass. At the bend in the fairway on the left side are two evergreen trees that stand as sentinels to keep golfers from cutting the corner too much. However, a well-placed tee shot just about anywhere on the fairway for a player like Jackson on this day would almost guarantee him at least a par or a bogey.

Jackson was the first to hit his tee shot from our group. We all saw the flight of the ball going toward the evergreen trees at the bend in the fairway. We were not quite sure, but we thought the ball hit the evergreen tree that was most lateral to the fairway. After everyone else had hit their shots, all of which landed on the fairway, we went searching for Jackson's ball. Jackson was the first one to the area, and he said his ball had landed in the grass between the two trees. In this location he had a good shot to the green.

Jackson hit his second shot from the grassy area between the two trees. Unfortunately, the ball was not hit well and only went a few yards forward. The rest of us saw that Jackson was obviously frustrated by his poor shot. To make matters worse, when Jackson squared up to hit his ball again, he noticed that the label on the ball was not his. He was playing a Titleist ball with three dots on it. The ball he had just hit was a Callaway ball. He called a penalty on himself for hitting the wrong ball.

There is a two stroke penalty for hitting the wrong ball. Our foursome then went back to the tree area to search for Jackson's ball. The ball was nowhere to be found, and collectively we assumed the ball remained lodged up in the evergreen tree. Jackson had to take an additional one stroke penalty for a lost ball.

After some consultation within our foursome we agreed where Jackson should drop his new ball, which he did. We could now see that Jackson was pretty frustrated with how things were turning out on this ninth hole. With his ego deflated and his emotions running high and most likely with his adrenaline levels also rising, Jackson hit his next shot well past the green into some trees between the last green and the clubhouse.

Jackson found his ball in a bad location just under the drip line branches of an evergreen tree. He could hit the ball but it wasn't going to be a very easy effort. Jackson gave his best try, but unfortunately he mishit the ball. It careened to the right and bounced into a sand bunker next to the green.

By now we saw that Jackson was beyond himself; his ability to concentrate had vanished. It took him two more shots to extricate his ball from the sand bunker. When his ball finally made it to the green, it was about 60 feet uphill from the flagstick. Jackson ended up taking four putts to finish the hole.

While hoping for his best score ever if he made a par 4 or a bogey five, Jackson settled for a score of 12, eight over par for the hole.

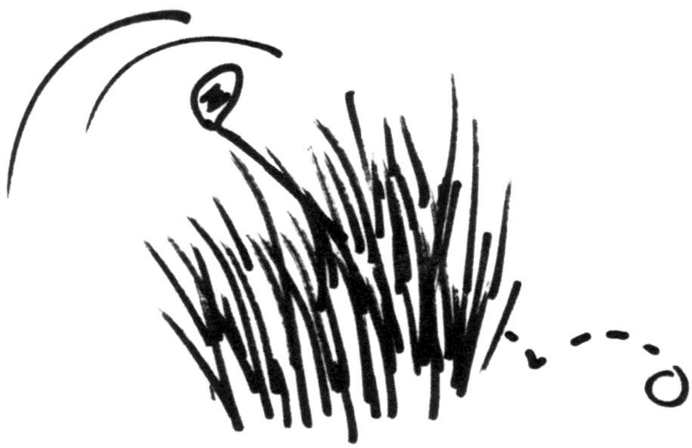

Afterward, I gave my condolences to Jackson. I told him that he could have hit that second shot out of the trees without calling a penalty on himself and none of us would been the wiser.

Jackson commented to me, “I would've known. You have to play by the rules. You have to play the ball where it lies. You know, golf is still just a game. It’s just a game.”

"If there's one thing golf commands above all else, is honesty."

Jack Nicklaus

Goose-in-One

The senior league golf tournaments have a shotgun start at 8 o'clock on Monday mornings. This means that all the teams go to an assigned hole and begin playing at the same time, i.e., 8 a.m. On this particular morning our foursome consisted of Lowell, Raymond, Bert, and me. We were assigned to start on the 12th hole which faces directly to the East. The morning was nearly cloudless, and the rising sun was intensely bright. The location of the sun was just a short distance above the trees on the horizon so that if I held my forearm horizontally near my forehead blocking the sunlight I could barely see the golfer teeing off. I was hopeful I could see the flight of the ball after it was struck. Otherwise, without blocking the sun, watching for the golf ball was almost impossible.

All teams are made up of A, B, C, and D level players according to their personal handicap scores. This was my first opportunity to play with Lowell and Raymond. I had played with Bert on several occasions before and knew that he was blind in one eye and had poor vision in the other eye. He was our foursome's D level player this day. After the first three members of our foursome hit their golf balls onto the fairway, it was Bert's turn.

The 12th tee box has a river-fed lake immediately to the right. This tee box is located near the turn of the adjacent fairway heading in the opposite direction. This lake frequently accommodates ducks and geese during the spring and summer months.

As Bert was preparing to tee off, we three remaining golfers took positions behind him, shielded our eyes from the sun, and hoped to watch his shot. We all commented about the difficulty looking toward the sun. Bert just laughed, as usual.

Just after Bert hit his driver, he said, "Where did it go?"

Lowell responded with, "I have no idea."

I said, "Sorry, I just didn't see a thing. When I looked up all I saw was the sun."

Raymond noted, "Bert, I saw it take off high into the sky, but then I lost it in the sun."

Despite three of us straining to see Bert's tee shot, we had no idea where it went. Bert, however, being familiar with his golf swing, was convinced that he had hit the ball well and that it went forward.

It just so happened that a good-sized flock of geese was flying toward the lake from the North across our fairway just as Bert was teeing off. We paid little attention to the birds since this was a common occurrence at the golf course.

Just a moment after Bert hit his shot I noticed a goose from the flying flock fall from the sky and lay lifeless on the fairway about a hundred yards away. I asked if anyone else saw the goose fall from the sky. Everyone except Bert saw the poor bird plummet to the ground.

As our foursome proceeded down the fairway and approached the dead-appearing goose lying on the fairway, the bird got up and slowly limped over to the lake to join his friends in the water. In the near vicinity of where the goose had landed, Raymond found Bert's golf ball. It appeared to us that the ball had indeed hit the goose in midair. He had scored a goose-in-one. We all had a good laugh as we continued down the fairway toward the green. As far as we could tell the goose that sustained the golf ball attack survived and was doing well swimming in the lake.

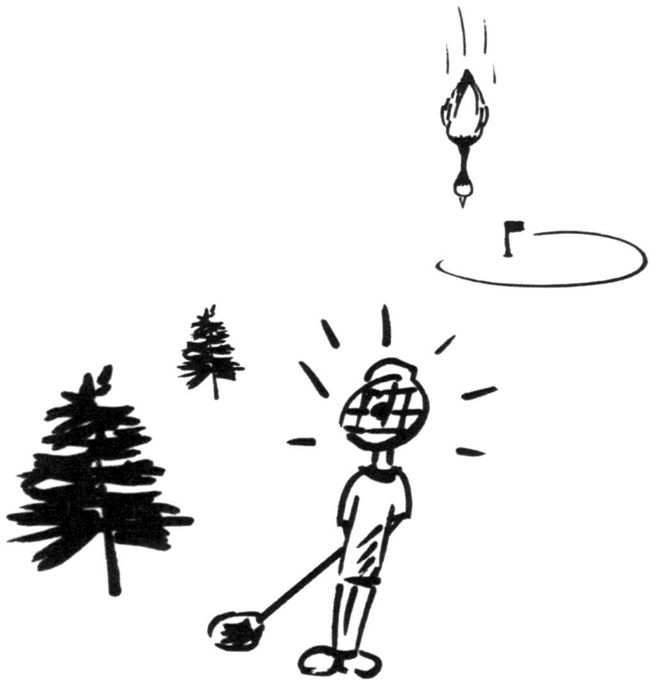

Bert hit his second shot poorly, and it bounced down the fairway about 150 hundred yards. He shanked his third shot to the right into a lake near the hole. Bert finally made it onto the green with his 5th shot. After hitting three putts Bert finally completed the hole, and his score of 8 was recorded. (A score of 8 is termed a snowman.) Bert exclaimed, “And it was a quality 8 to boot!”

I mentioned to Bert that not too many golfers can profess to have scored a snowman AND a goose-in-one on the same hole.

Nose Plug

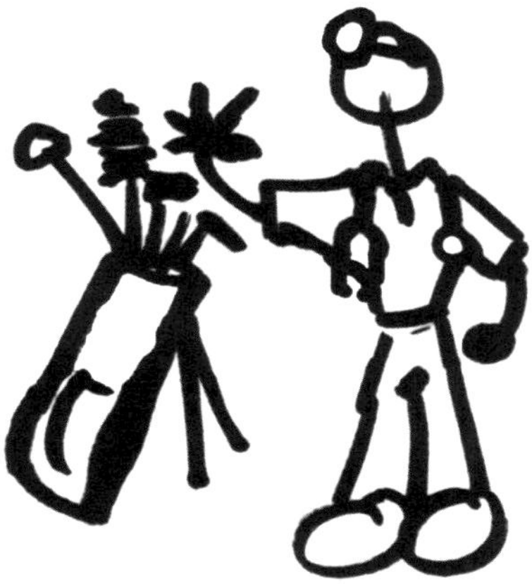

Frank and Marjorie lived in Central Florida. One summer, because it was unbearably hot and humid in Florida, they decided to finally visit some friends and relatives in Montana. In the two weeks before coming to Billings, the pair had stayed in the high mountain communities of Big Sky and Red Lodge. They stopped in Billings as their last Montana stop before returning to Florida.

Before going home, Frank and Marjorie decided to play golf one day in Billings. I guess they truly enjoyed playing golf since they had played seven days out of the previous fourteen days while in Montana. They were on the driving range warming up to play when I arrived. It just so happened that the pair and I were the only golfers on the driving range at that time.

As I was about ready to pull out my first golf club from my bag, I heard Marjorie cry out, “Oh Frank, not again!”

This commotion certainly caught my attention. As I turned around to see what's going on, I saw Marjorie on her hands and knees with blood streaming out of her nose. She was not holding her nose or attempting to stop the bleeding in any way. She was just allowing the blood to run. Frank was rubbing the back of her neck and saying some comforting words.

I asked if I could be of assistance. I advised the pair that I was a physician.

Frank complained that the air in Montana was so dry compared to the air in Florida; Marjorie was having a lot of nosebleeds.

I asked him what they had done in the past few weeks to stop the bleeding.

Frank told me that they just let the blood run from his wife’s nose for a while; it always stopped.

I asked if Marjorie had been sick or if she had some major disease.

Marjorie said she was healthy as a horse.

I asked if she had been taking any medicines that I should know about.

Marjorie replied that the only medicine she had been using was some eyedrops because she appeared to have allergies in Montana also. Her eyes had been red and irritated their entire trip.

I got Marjorie to sit up straight, and I noticed blood coming only from the right side of her nose. I showed her where to place her thumb and index finger to put pressure on the soft part of her nose to stop the bleeding. I asked her to squeeze hard for five minutes by the clock.

Frank said he would make sure the time was right.

I asked them if Marjorie had been using any other medicines for her allergies.

Frank said, "Marjorie has only been using the eyedrops we already mentioned and a Chapstick to moisten her parched lips."

As Marjorie was pinching her nose and her husband being the official timer, I told them I would be right back. I went into the clubhouse and asked the club pro if he had an emergency kit.

He did. The man retrieved a small white plastic case that had an emergency label on it.

Inside the kit I found a box of rolled gauze. I told the pro that I would pay him back.

He wanted to know what was going on.

I told him there was a woman on the driving range who had a nosebleed.

The pro wanted to know if it was the man and woman visiting from Florida having the problems.

When I commented that indeed it was them, he told me that the course wasn't very busy for a while. He would get them out to play as soon as they were ready.

Upon returning to the driving range, I found Marjorie still holding your nose. The bleeding appeared to have stopped. Marjorie was more concerned about the blood all over her new white golfing shirt than she was about the possibility of bleeding to death.

I asked Frank if he would please give me his Chapstick. He promptly pulled it out of his pocket and handed it to me. I then asked him if he could find the eyedrops that Marjorie had been using if they were readily available. He located a bottle of Visine eyedrops in Marjorie's purse.

As I was gathering these materials, I was explaining to the pair from where the bleeding was most likely coming, that is, the fragile septum membrane in her nose. All I had to do was find a way to shrink the blood vessels in her nose and to moisturize the membrane so it wouldn't bleed anymore. In this process, I pulled out a good length of gauze from the box of gauze I took from the club pro and cut it with a knife that I retrieved from my golf bag. I saturated the gauze with the Visine, which I knew contained a blood vessel constrictor. Then I smeared most of the contents of the Chapstick onto the gauze. The primary ingredient in the Chapstick is petroleum jelly which would lubricate the nose.

Using a golf tee, I tightly packed the medicated piece of gauze into the right side of Marjorie's nose. Presto! The bleeding problem was resolved.

I asked Marjorie and Frank to wait in their golf cart for a few minutes to make sure that the bleeding was totally under control and for me to be sure that all the decongestant I put into Marjorie's nose did not produce an adverse effect.

After perhaps 10 more minutes and no more new bleeding occurring, I asked Marjorie to smear the remaining portion of the Chapstick into the left side of her nose for lubrication.

I asked Marjorie to keep the plug in her nose for at least six hours more. Afterward, she could apply some saline nasal spray and more Vaseline in her nose as she needed.

The pair wanted to pay me something for my emergency services. Frank asked how much I charged for an emergency visit to a driving range at a golf course on a beautiful August afternoon on my day off.

I just laughed and smiled. I replied that I was just an old retired country doc doing what I have always done. I encouraged the pair to have a good time playing golf in Montana.

"The more I work and practice,
the luckier I seem to get."
Gary Player

A Good Deal

Two friends from Montana accompanied Kay, my wife, and me when we visited the Orlando, Florida, area one year in the early fall. After spending a few days at the Disney World theme parks, we decided that we would play golf. Trying to be a conscientious tourist, I tried to make sure I found a good deal for golfing in one of the many promotional magazines that were available. In one magazine I found a promotion for the Kissimmee Golf Club in Kissimmee, Florida. The promotional coupon stated, "A round of golf with a cart and a sleeve of balls for $40."

I thought this was a good deal so we discussed the promotion and decided to call the golf course for a tee time to determine if the offer was legitimate.

I telephoned the Kissimmee Golf Club at the phone number listed on the advertisement, I told man who answered the phone that I had seen the advertisement in a magazine, and asked him if the promotion was still available.

The man replied, "No, sir, that promotion is no longer current." He then went on to explain that with the new promotion we could play a round of golf with a cart and have lunch for a fee of $25 each. A sleeve of balls was no longer a part of the promotion.

I asked the man, "What's the catch?"

The fellow replied, "There is no catch, sir."

I thought this was a little bit too good to be true. I asked the fellow, "What does lunch actually include? Is it a hot dog and a bag of chips at the turn or what?"

The fellow chuckled a bit and said, "No sir, we have a full-service snack bar. Each day we have at least six items to choose from that are available to our guests."

I asked the man to sign us up for four players at 10 a.m. the next morning.

Our group arrived a little bit early so we could see the course and warm-up. I walked up to the counter in the pro shop, gave my name to the young man behind the counter, and told him that we had a tee time at 10 o'clock. I asked him if the promotion that I called about the day before was still $25 dollars for golf, a cart, and lunch.

The young man said, “No sir, that promotion changed today.”

Worrying that we have been duped by some false advertising, I asked the young pro if there was a promotion for the day.

He said, “You're the guy from Montana I talked to yesterday aren't you?”

I replied, “Yes. We’re all from Montana.”

The young man smiled again and told us that the new promotion, as of that morning, was $25 for a round of golf with a cart, lunch at the snack bar, and a free golf shirt from the three racks behind me.

I asked the fellow if he was kidding me.

He told us that the golf club had a new boss from Pennsylvania who owned some coal mines. The new owner came down to the Kissimmee Golf Club, which apparently was one of four golf courses the man had acquired in the Orlando area, looked it over with his own groundskeeper, and wanted to make some changes. In the process the new boss instructed the employees in the pro shop to clear out all the clothing inventory. So that's just what they were doing.

Hearing the words “free shirts,” the two ladies were on those clothes racks faster than bees go to honey. Within moments, Kay was holding up a shirt on my back to see if it would fit. She said, “These things retail for

$60!" While Kay was locating the best colored shirt for herself and me, I paid our fees at the counter. Kay later gifted her shirt to me.

Before we went to get our golf cart and our clubs, the four of us checked out the cafe and its offerings for the day. The six available free lunch meals included a fried shrimp basket, fish and chips, hamburger and fries, Cobb salad, tuna sandwich with chips, and a hot dog with fries. Drinks were extra. We were all amazed at the value.

Our group had a marvelous outing playing golf. The Kissimmee Golf Club proved to be an adequately maintained public course with greens that were quite good. As we were leaving the eighteenth green and returning to the clubhouse, there was a small sign by the cart path that that read, "Play another round of golf for only $9."

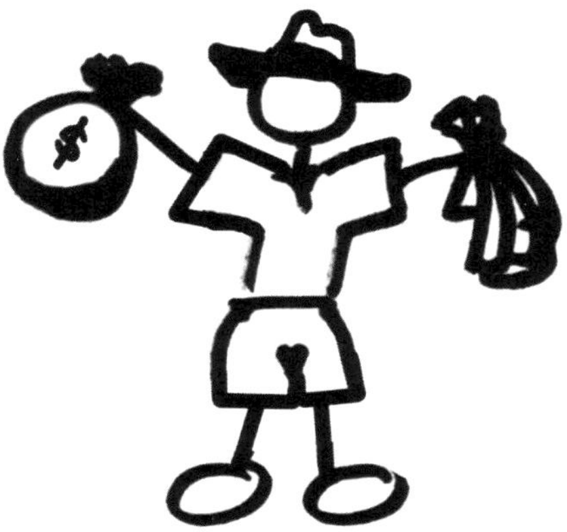

I thought we had found a small gold mine in the golf mecca of Florida. I figured that we had each received at least $120 worth of goods and services for $25. We decided right then that we would have to return the next day to play again.

When we returned the next day, the shirt promotion was over because all the shirts were gone! Big surprise! However, to play golf with a cart and to have lunch at the snack bar still cost only $25.

On multiple occasions when I wore one of my Kissimmee Golf Club labeled shirts playing senior league golf, someone would come up to me, look at the logo on my shirt, and say, "Kiss me?"

Having some fun with the golfer, I would tell him, "Not now, but maybe later."

Seeing the golfer's reaction to my retort was usually priceless. I would then tell them the story of how I got a free shirt on vacation in Florida.

A Practical Joke

It was my second year of senior golf league participation and actually my second year of trying to play golf well. Gradually, I was becoming familiar with some of the names and faces of the nearly 100 seniors who played in the league. On this particular day the game was a modified scramble format with a rule that each player had to provide at least one drive from the tee box during the nine-hole game except for the par three holes. Our foursome started on the first hole of the second nine holes (hole number 10).

I was about fifteen years or more younger than the other members of our foursome. Somehow, they all knew that I could hit the ball relatively far and straight. Therefore, on the first hole, which was a par five, we used up a shorter drive that was in the fairway but only about 130 yards away. With two quality shots from the fairway and a magnificent long putt from one of the guys, our team managed to score a 4, a birdie, on this hole.

The next hole was a par 4 and almost 400 yards. It was rated as the hardest hole on the course. Again, our team used a drive in the fairway that was not very far, but was well-placed in the center of the fairway. We managed to have two more good shots from the fairway to reach the green. The ball settled perhaps ten feet above the flagstick. A superb long downhill putt preserved our team's par for the hole.

Our third hole was a par 4 and again almost 400 yards. There was a lake located to the right and partially in front of the green. This time, however, the wind was at our backs which gave our drives a bit of a boost. We chose a ball that was driven onto the fairway and about 170 yards from the center of the green for our second shot. We noticed that the flagstick was located near the front of the large green and was only about 150 yards away. One of our team members used his fairway wood to hit a ball that carried only about 100 yards in the air but continued to roll onto the green. Another magnificent putt gave our team another birdie. After three holes our team was 2 strokes under par.

The next hole was a par three and each member of the foursome had to hit his own ball by the rules of the game. Our team came away with a par.

The 14th hole is only 300 yards by official measurement. It has a severe dogleg left alignment with the midpoint being about 150 yards from the tee box. The hole also has a lake between the tee box and the green on the left side of the fairway. If the intrepid golfer felt so inclined, a drive that carried in the air approximately 200 yards would place the ball in the middle of the fairway somewhere between the green and 80 yards away depending upon the quality of the drive.

I knew that none of the older three members of our foursome had hit a ball over 150 yards all day. Despite this reality, the first golfer got up and said, "I'm going for it!" Aiming directly over the lake, his ball landed approximately ten yards into the lake.

The second golfer teed up his golf ball and, looking at his friend who had just hit his ball into the lake said, "What a weakling. Let me show you how it's done." With his pre-shot setup this golfer waggled a bit with his driver behind the ball before making a mighty swing. His golf ball flew straight and true into the middle of the lake perhaps a few feet farther than his friend. He exited the tee box appearing disgusted as his friends razzed his shot.

The third golfer walked to the tee box, looked at his friends, and exclaimed, "I'll show you how it's done boys!"

He then hit a ball that bounced on the ground about 100 yards after takeoff, bounced several times in the rough, and then rolled weakly into the lake. He too was razzed by his friends.

As I walked to the tee box I looked at my three teammates who, with big smiles on their faces and almost in unison said, "Jim, looks like we could use a ball in the fairway." Then they laughed. The three older guys had connived to have some fun with the youngster on their

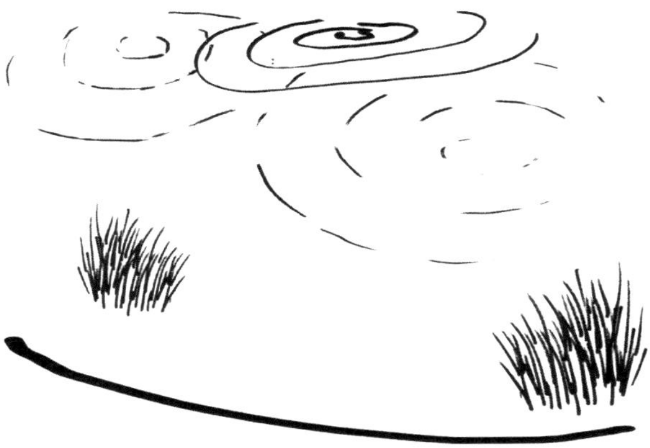

team. That was me.

Fortunately, I did not succumb to the pressure and hit a ball that landed in the middle of the fairway about 100 yards away from the green. With another good fairway-to-green shot from one of the other players and another excellent putt, our team scored a birdie 3.

Our team went on to score well enough to take first place for the day. We had a good time, no one suffered an injury, and we all earned more pro shop credit.

The old guys played a good joke on their younger partner to perfection.

It could not have been a better day!

Three Amigos

It was a Wednesday morning at 8:00 on the 10th tee box at Yegen Golf Club. The golf pro had assigned me to play with three gentlemen who were already on the tee box and called out on the loudspeaker to notify them that I would be joining them. It was a beautiful sunny morning with no wind and few clouds. I thought to myself that it was a marvelous day to play golf. As I walked to the 10th tee box I saw three golfers ready to play. They all welcomed me to join them and introduced themselves as Randall, Lauren, and Marvin. They told me that they had already played, and it was my turn. Without warming up, I took a few swings with my 3-wood and hit the ball down the fairway.

As we started walking down the fairway, the three golfers spoke freely among themselves. I noticed that Randall had a large bruise on the left side of his face, but I was reluctant to ask him how it occurred. Marvin, on the other hand, asked Randall, “Hey Randall, tell us about the bruise on your face.”

Randall let us know that his wife Helen had an episode while they were making supper the night before. He related that while he was making their evening meal on the stove his wife picked up a frying pan and hit him on the side of his face. She thought he was an intruder. Randall noted that he thought Helen's Alzheimer's disease was getting worse and he may have to put her in a nursing care facility pretty soon. In fact, he was meeting with the people from the nursing home that day.

Randall then asked Lauren about his sore arm. I then noticed a wrist splint on the man’s left arm. As I understood the conversation, Lauren’s wife Marjorie had significant dementia also. Lauren noted that his left wrist injury was mending as well as could be expected. Apparently, Marjorie had an episode of severe confusion about two weeks before that became violent. In the process of restraining her with the help of paramedics, Lauren sustained a significant injury to his wrist. After his wife spent a few days in the hospital for a psychiatric evaluation, Lauren took her home to continue caring for her. He also voiced that it wouldn't be long before his wife would have to be placed in a memory care facility.

Marvin was the silent, quiet man of the three golfers. When Lauren asked him how his wife Joyce was doing, Marvin just said, “Joyce is really bad.” He continued to say that he completed the paperwork to get his wife placed in the Alzheimer's wing in the nursing home. He was just waiting for a spot to open up for her. Marvin uttered that he could no longer care for Joyce at home. Marvin interjected that he found his wife walking down the street with only her nightgown on early the previous morning when it was only 40°. He said he was unable to sleep for fear of what she would do in the house or, perhaps even worse, what would happen to her when she went off wondering.

As we continued playing nine holes of golf that morning, I learned that these three gentlemen were indeed heroes to their wives; their wives would never know it because of their dementias. As the three men chatted I learned that twice a week they got together at 8 o'clock in the morning to play golf. It was only during these times of the week that the men did not provide 24-hour care for their spouses. Each man talked about the logistics of getting someone who was familiar with and understanding of dementia patients to care for their spouse just for a few hours so he could get to the golf course. Having spent my life in medicine and observing people, it appeared to me that the three men were near physical and emotional exhaustion. Playing golf two times a week was this trio's only reprieve from their daily arduous duties taking care of their spouses; the only times they could really communicate with friends who actually understood and appreciated their predicaments.

These men did not play any special golf games. They did not keep their individual scores. They just walked, talked, and played golf together.

As we were finishing up playing nine holes of golf that morning, I told the men that they reminded me of the three musketeers, "All for one and one for all."

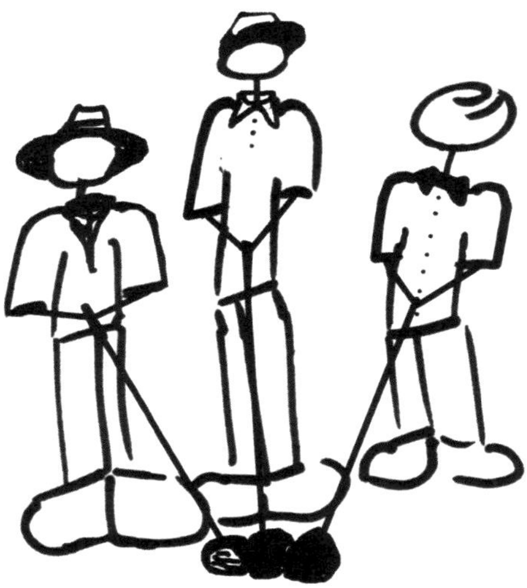

They agreed with me.

We all shook hands, the three men patted each other on their backs, wished each other well, and then each one returned to their respective homes to be trusted caregivers for their spouses.

Within the Leather

One day when the golf course appeared to be relatively free of golfers, I was playing a round of golf by myself at my usual brisk pace. When I got to the tee box of the par 3 third hole, I saw a threesome in front of me on the fairway about ready to hit their second shots toward the green. I noticed one of the golfers was quite large. I witnessed him get into the golf cart on the right side and the cart appeared to instantly list to that side. By the time I finished playing the hole, the threesome was approaching the next tee box.

I reached the next tee box just after the second player had played his shot. After the third player finished his tee shot, one of the gentlemen asked me to join them because they were not very fast players and the group in front of them was not playing briskly either.

I agreed.

After our introductions on the tee box, I hit my shot on the par five hole. I soon appreciated that the gentlemen were having a lot of fun with the heavyset fellow. Having taken care of a lot of overweight individuals during my years of medicine, I guesstimated that this massive man weighed somewhere between 400 and 450 pounds. His physique reminded me of a large bowling pin stuck on top of two toothpicks. I figured his waist must be 60 inches or more in circumference.

As we made our way toward the green I heard a considerable amount of banter among the three golfers. It seemed to me that they had some sort of a wagering game among themselves, and they appeared to be having a wonderful time doing it.

As we approached the large green on this par five hole we noticed that the flagstick placement was directly in the center of the green. Eventually, we were ready to putt. I was on the green in three shots about 15 feet away from the flagstick. Two of the other golfers were on the green in five shots some distance from the flag. The overweight man's golf ball was lying at five shots just off the green a few yards.

The big man took out his club and said, "Watch this boys." He then proceeded to chip his ball relatively close to the hole. He then asked, "Is it good?"

One of his companions said, "Jonathon, you know the ball has to be within the leather."

Being new to the game I did not know what 'within the leather' meant, so I watched and learned.

The overweight golfer proceeded to remove his belt and stretch it from the hole to his golf ball, a distance of about 5 feet I surmised. His ball was just 'inside the leather,' the length of his leather belt.

I was amazed initially at the length of the man's belt and then at his ingenuity to use his belt as a measuring tool.

One of his playing partners asked the big fellow what he thought he was doing. He explained to the overweight man that he was supposed to measure the distance with his putter. The ball on the putting surface had to be within the distance from the flagstick to the leather on the putter's grip to be counted as a "gimmee" (give me) putt.

The overweight man responded with, "My putter's grip is not leather! The only leather I have on me is my belt, so I used it."

All three players had a good-natured laugh and the companion players gave their heavyset friend credit for a putt that was 'within the leather.' However, they cautioned him that he only got to use the belt trick once. NEVER AGAIN!

We all had a good laugh on the way to the next tee box.

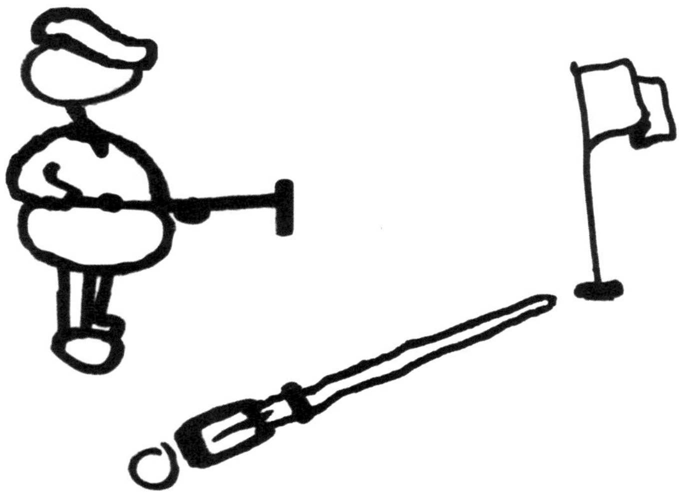

"Have you ever noticed? Anybody going slower than you is an idiot, and anyone going faster than you is a maniac."

Unknown

Lucky 7

The 13th hole is a 135-yard par 3. To the right of the tee area is a small lake that is fed by irrigation water from the Yellowstone River. To the left of the tee box is an asphalt walkway and an out-of-bounds barbed-wire fence which continues the entire length of the hole. The backside of the green has sand bunkers that welcome an overzealous shot followed by another out-of-bounds barbed-wire fence.

Herbert was the first of our foursome to tee off this particular morning. He was also our highest handicap player. Herbert lined up to take a shot, made an unorthodox swing at the ball, and shanked the ball directly into the lake on the right.

After quietly uttering a few colorful metaphors, Herbert lined up again to take a second shot. Since he had to take a penalty stroke for losing a ball in water, this shot would count as number 3. Again, Herbert aligned himself to hit the ball. This time, however, he aimed his body a little bit farther left. Unfortunately, Herbert pointed the face of his golf club directly at the flagstick. This alignment almost invites a slicing shot to the right. He hit the ball and, as one would expect with his alignment, the ball curved even farther into the lake on the right. The ducks swimming in the lake did not move because apparently golf balls flying past them was a frequent occurrence on this lake.

One of the other golfers suggested that Herbert just drop his ball in a drop zone closer to the green. However, it had now become a matter of man versus golf ball. After exclaiming a few more profanities out loud, Herbert lined up to hit his next shot which would now be counted as his 5th shot. Again, Herbert aligned the face of his golf club to be square with the flagstick. This time he aimed his feet even farther left and he swung his golf club even harder. As I expected, his 5th shot curved more severely to the right. This ball skipped on the water and came to rest on the beach on the far edge of the lake.

One of the other golfers asked Herbert if he had seen the movie *Tin Cup* where the golfer played by Kevin Costner kept hitting a ball over the lake until the ball went into the hole.

Herbert yelled back, "Yeh, yeh, I get it!"

His friend and fellow golfer suggested that Herbert aim his golf club, not his feet, a little bit farther left.

Herbert told him that he would do just that.

Unfortunately, when Herbert aimed his golf club a little bit farther to the left of the flagstick he did not change his stance which was aimed directly left at the out-of-bounds area. When he struck the ball this time, which was now his 7th shot on this hole, the ball took off like a rocket in a straight line. It quickly passed over the out-of-bounds wire fence, over the asphalt walkway, and struck a tall wooden fence about halfway between the tee box and the green. The ball then careened off the fence, flew high into the air, and landed on the green about 3 feet above the flagstick.

Herbert raised his arms in triumph, let out a hoot, and exclaimed, "Now that's what I'm talking about!"

Our entire group laughed out loud.

Herbert made it to the green on a par 3 hole with just 7 shots! He then three putted for a 10!

One of the guys quipped, "Nice 10 Herbie."

Herbert replied, "Thanks guys!"

We then traversed the short distance to the next tee box.

To me, Herbie certainly was a sure-fire case for patient persistence. Another golf lesson for me.

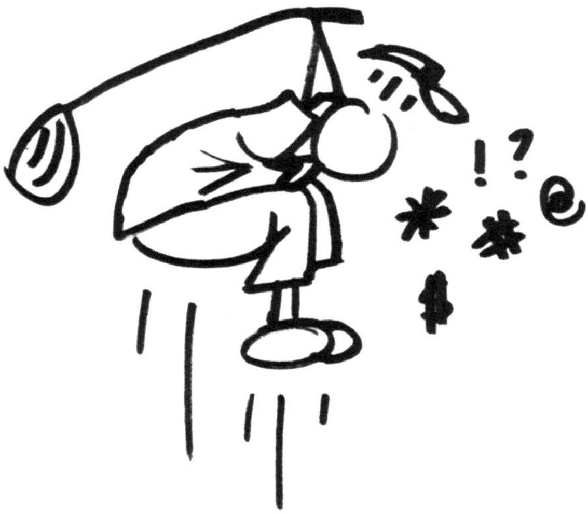

"It's about hitting the ball in the center of the club face and hitting it hard."

Bubba Watson

Doc, Ya got a Minute

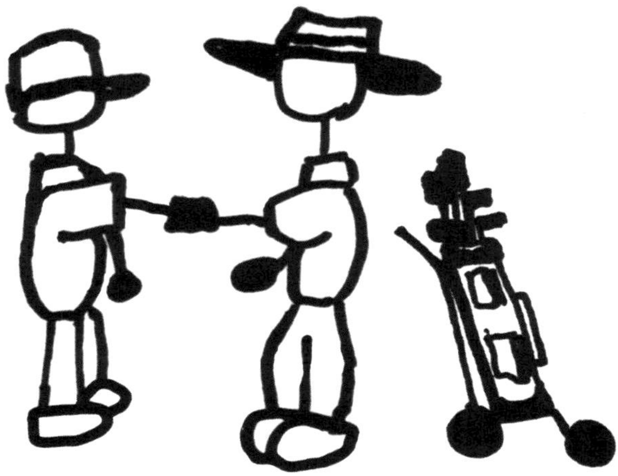

I was in the parking lot of the golf course putting my clubs away after our senior league event was completed for the day. At the time I was about sixty-five years old. Another golfer came by my pickup truck, stopped his car, and got out to talk to me. He said something like, "Hello, my name is Bertram. You don't know me, but I understand that you're a doctor."

I told a man that I was indeed a physician.

He then asked, "Do you have some time? Would you mind if I asked you a medical question?"

I told the man that I would be glad to answer his questions as well as I could. I asked him how I might help.

Bertram asked me what kind of doctor I was.

As usual, I told him that I was one of the last of the Mohicans. That is, I was a country doc in the boondocks mostly in Montana who got to do and see a lot of things. I was also an instructor in medicine for over thirty years.

The man asked me if I could give him a second opinion about something.

I told him that I would be glad to tell him anything that I knew about a topic in medicine. If I did not know the answer, I offered to find more information for him. Besides, I told him the consultation was free since I was no longer in active practice.

Bertram told me that he had just gone to his doctor the day before and was told that he had leukemia. According to this man his physician said there was nothing that needed to be done.

I asked Bertram, "How old are you?"

"Seventy-seven," was his reply.

I asked him why he went to see the doctor in the first place. I questioned if he was sick.

Bertram explained that he was feeling fine. His wife suggested that he should see a doctor because he was indeed getting older; something might need to be fixed, and besides their insurance paid for the doctor visit for free.

I asked the man how old he thought he would be when he died.

He told me he really had not thought about it. He always figured that mother nature would take its course, and one day he would just keel over dead.

Since Bertram was older than me by almost a decade, I informed him that when he was born his life expectancy was only 60 years. Therefore, in some respects and statistically speaking, he should consider himself fortunate since he should have been dead seventeen years before.

Bertram gazed at me in bewilderment.

I continued to tell Bertram that since he was not sick and since he could have had this "leukemia" for an unknown period of time, I would agree with his doctor's suggestion that nothing be done just because of his age.

Bertram asked me, "But he said I had leukemia. Won't that kill me?"

I suggested to Bertram that my suspicion was that he had a chronic disease such as chronic lymphocytic leukemia, or CLL, which at his age was a wait and watch disorder. He may have had the disease for years and did not know it. I also told him that at his age a course of chemotherapy for the leukemia might be worse than the disease itself.

Bertram told me that he remembered that his doctor did say something about CLL.

I asked Bertram if he had a computer.

He said that he did.

I suggested that he first call his doctor's office to confirm his diagnosis. Then he could find articles about the disease on the internet or at the public library before scheduling another face-to-face discussion with his doctor about his diagnosis.

Finally, I encouraged Bertram to go out and shoot his age on the golf course.

Not too many days later Bertram came up to me about 7:30 in the morning during our senior golf league warm-up and told me that he had followed my advice. He had obtained his diagnosis from his doctor's office, he checked out what he could find and understand on the internet, and then took that information to his doctor. He told me that he and his doctor had a good discussion about his 'leukemia' which was indeed chronic lymphocytic leukemia or CLL. Bertram told me that the doctor said pretty much what I told him with my impromptu consultation in the parking lot. He thanked me for my time and gave me his best wishes to play well.

On this particular day I did score well. I scored my age, 68, my best score ever. Unfortunately, our team score was not good enough to place in the top three; we did not receive any of those coveted pro shop credits.

It has now been about three years since I first saw Bertram in the parking lot. He is now over 80, he appears well for his age, and he did not receive any treatment for his chronic leukemia. Unfortunately, his golf game has not improved with time. Nonetheless, he still enjoys the game of golf and trying to score his age!

The Warmup

The Toka Sticks golf course in Mesa, Arizona was started around 1950 by the United States Air Force to provide a recreational facility for those stationed at the Williams Air Force Base. In the early 1990s the operation of the 18-hole golf course was taken over by the Gila River Indian community and promoted as a private golf course. Since then the golf course has matured and has become one of the most popular and one of the best value golf facilities in the Phoenix area.

My wife Kay and I visited some friends in the Mesa area one winter. Beside sightseeing in the Phoenix area, our friends took us to the Toga Sticks golf course one morning for a relaxing round of golf.

While my wife and friends were paying the fees for us to play and checking out the clothing bargains in the clubhouse, I ventured over to the driving range to stretch and warm up. Strange as it may seem the older I get the more I need to stretch and warm-up before I play.

The Toka Sticks driving range had only eight or so spaces for golfers to hit balls while warming up to play. Consequently, it was almost impossible not to see and hear what the other players on the driving range were saying and doing.

As I was stretching before I hit my first shot, I observed a woman to my left who was about ready to hit her golf ball. The woman made a mighty swing at her ball, and during the completion of her swing, she released her golf club at shoulder level sending the club flying high into the air and landing behind her about 20 yards. She let out a loud “Whoa” as she was completing her swing.

The mortified woman looked at me and said, “Did anybody see where it went?”

Having observed the entire episode, I told the woman that her ball was still sitting on the tee.

The woman then responded, “No, I meant where did my golf club go?”

I pointed my finger behind her and told the woman that the golf club flew high in the air and landed directly behind her about 20 yards away.

The woman spun around, saw her golf club, and strutted to that area looking side to side to see if anyone else saw her mishap. She was wide-eyed and appeared disgusted.

When she returned to the tee box she commented to me, “You know, it is just so hard to hold a golf club with long finger nails!”

I didn’t say a word.

The woman gathered her wits, took another stance beside her golf ball, waggled her golf club in preparation for her next attempt, and made a mighty swing at her teed-up golf ball. She twisted, contorted, and spun her body on her left leg 360 ° without the club coming close to the ball. Whiff!

On her third try the woman missed her golf ball easily by 12 inches. Whiff again.

I could see that the lady was becoming exasperated. On the fourth attempt she fixed her eyes intently on her ball, stiffened her wrists and her elbows, clenched her jaws, and swung her club much easier. Eureka, she hit the it. The ball bounced only a few feet in front of her, but she did hit the ball. Aha, progress!

With her fifth attempt, the woman was able to hit the golf ball into the air, finally.

With a few subsequent shots, the woman’s golf balls sailed forward not very far, but forward, without any problems. Her golf clubs did not exit from her hands again.

As her golfing companion came to pick her up with a golf cart, I wished the woman luck.

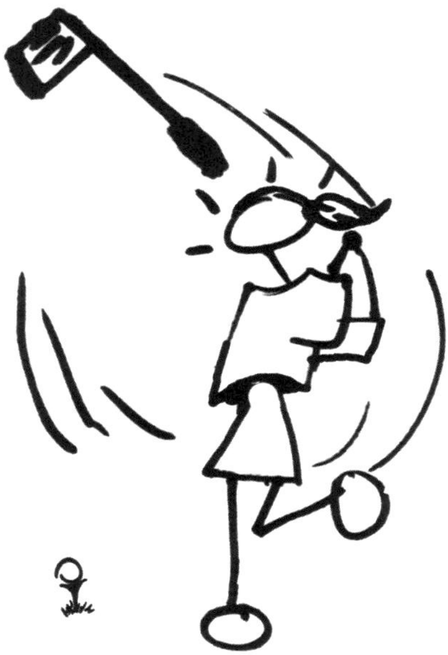

"I know I am getting better at golf because
I am hitting fewer spectators."
Gerald R. Ford

The Long Jumper

I had been playing with the senior league golf for only a few months when I was paired with three golfers more senior in age to me for the morning's game. Our foursome started the day on the 7th hole which is a straight par 5 about 460 yards long. The distance between our teeing area and the most forward tee box, also affectionately called the ladies' tee box, is about 70 yards. An irrigation ditch, which is perhaps 2 feet wide at the most, traverses between the two tee boxes. During the spring and summer months the ditch fills with water to the depth of at most one and a half feet. The water fills the ponds and lakes on the golf course and provides water for irrigating the remaining areas of the golf course.

Norman, a small gentleman in his mid-80s, was the first of our foursome to hit his tee shot. He was the high handicap player for our group, but he refused to use the forward, or ladies', tee box. Using the forward tee box is a courtesy for those players who own quite high handicaps or who are over 80 years old.

After a mighty swing Norman's driver slammed into the earth behind his teed-up golf ball. The ball then hit the ground about 3 inches in front of the tee before it bounced high into the air. It carried about 20 yards before falling into the deep grass in front of the irrigation ditch. Norman walked off to sit in his golf cart while we remaining three players hit our shots.

Norman then got out of his golf cart and proclaimed his first ball was an unplayable lie. He was going to take a one-stroke penalty and hit another tee shot. Before hitting his ball Norman proclaimed, "Now hitting three."

This time Norman placed his ball a little higher on a tee. After taking a few practice swings with his driver,

Norman made another hefty swing at his ball. This time his club went under the ball before striking it. The ball sailed high into the sky and landed on the other side of the irrigation ditch in plain view, but about 10 yards short of the ladies' tee box. After saying a few special words to the golf gods, Norman encouraged the rest of us to go on ahead while he picked up his ball in front of the irrigation ditch.

After finding his ball in the deep grass about 10 yards short of the irrigation ditch and seeing his other golf ball just on the other side of the ditch behind the ladies' tee box, Norman decided to hop the ditch instead of walking around to the cart path which went over the ditch irrigation culvert ten yards away from him.

My back was turned when I heard a "sploosh." As I turned around, I saw Norman looking dejected and disgusted standing in the middle of the irrigation ditch knee deep in water. He looked totally dumbfounded. He looked at the three of us and exclaimed, "And to think in track I used to be a long jumper!"

The sight of this old fellow standing in an irrigation ditch up to his knees in water was priceless and made us all laugh, including Norman. Not only had he hurt his pride, but also he had just ruined his brand-new golf shoes. After one of the other golfers helped Norman out of the ditch, he walked over to his second golf ball with his new shoes sloshing with water the entire way.

Norman picked out a golf club from his bag on the golf cart and hit a nice fourth shot down the fairway. As he was getting into his golf cart, one of the other members of the foursome and obviously one of his good friends said to him, "Hey Norm, you didn't make it to the ladies' tee box not once but twice on the same hole. You know what that means don't you?"

Before we knew it, Norman turned around to his friend and dropped his pants. He then said, "Now we're even!" (I assumed this was some sort of payback from a previous incident.)

His two friends had a great laugh at Norman's expense. I was little bit shocked that someone would drop his pants and moon his playing companions on the golf course.

Before Norman played his next shot he mumbled to himself, "I dubbed two drives on the SAME hole, I couldn't jump a one-foot ditch, I ruined my brand-new golf shoes, and I showed my butt to God and all his creatures. What else can I do wrong today?"

Fortunately for Norman, nothing else bad happened to him the rest of this golf round.

After our group finished the last hole and I again shook the hands of my three playing partners, I thanked them for their lessons of the day.

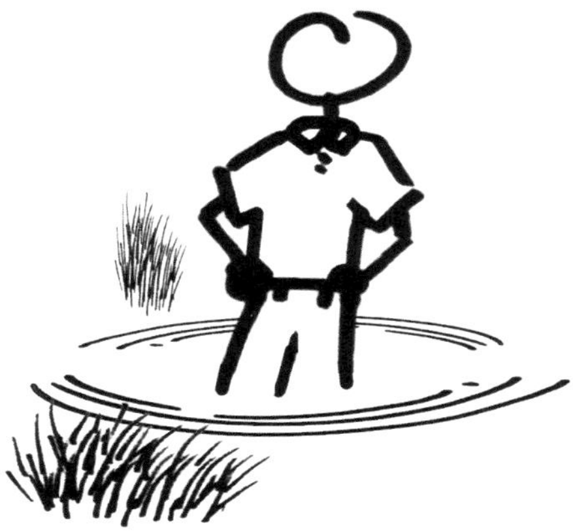

"I have a tip that can take five strokes off anyone's game: It's called an eraser."
Arnold Palmer

Coed Golfing

Men and women golfers at our golf course have their respective golf leagues for seniors and non-seniors. Our senior league plays on Monday mornings while the women play in their league on Tuesday mornings. When a national holiday occurs on a Monday, our senior league does not host an event. The women graciously allow the senior men golfers to join them for a fun co-educational scramble on their regular Tuesday morning league. Personally, I always found this to be a most enjoyable time. However, I came to realize that some of my male colleagues did not want to play with women golfers under any circumstances. I have been told by some of the women golfers that they felt intimidated or belittled by the men. Therefore, they would not play golf with them even if it was supposed to be a fun event.

During my first year playing senior league golf, I had the opportunity to play in my very first coed golf scramble on the Tuesday after the Memorial Day holiday. I must admit that I had a marvelous time. Carol, the female golfer in our contingent, proved to be a magnificent putter and short game player.

I really don't remember if our team scored well enough to win any pro shop credits, but the name of the game was to have a good time, and I did.

When the scramble was over, I walked by Carol in the parking lot as she was loading her equipment into the back of her vehicle. Again, I congratulated her. I told her I had a wonderful time playing with her on our team.

She echoed the same to me in return. She then asked me, "Do you mind if I ask you a medical question? This is about a friend of mine."

I told Carol that I would be glad to let her know what I knew and give her an unofficial opinion since I was not her physician.

Carol said her friend was diagnosed with breast cancer a few days before and she was worried. Carol wanted to know how long her friend was going to live.

I told Carol that there are many variations with breast cancer just as there are with any cancer. A prognosis depended upon many factors including the type of cancer, how aggressive the cancer cells were, and how much the tumor had spread. Having been in this scenario many times before, I asked Carol, "Is your friend you?"

I could see her eyes becoming tearful, and she just nodded her head affirmatively without saying a word.

Trying to be helpful and hopefully giving her the best answer I could, I asked Carol if she knew anything more about her tumor. I asked her if she remembered anything about what her doctor told her.

She said she had a screening mammogram done which showed a small breast cancer that was about 1 millimeter in size. She recalled the doctor telling her the tumor was stage 0. After that, she said her mind went blank. She really did not recall much more of what the doctor said after he mentioned she had a "breast cancer." She told me that panic set in. She became a total basket case. Carol did recall, however, that the doctor wanted to have a biopsy done within a week or so.

I asked the woman her age.

She told me, "I am 68 years old."

I told her that stage 0 breast cancer is the best kind to have. I mentioned that after she had a breast biopsy, which in my experience probably could be done with a needle because it was so small, her doctor may want her to receive some radiation treatments. I reinforced the idea that patients with stage 0 tumors that were not aggressive frequently did not receive any chemotherapy. I told her I would probably bet my house on her being around to play golf for least another 10 years, and the chance for dying from breast tumor were almost 0.

Carol asked, “Are you serious? Or are you just trying to make me feel good?”

I told her that I had recently written a book about my experiences as a family doctor, and breast cancer was one of topics in the book. I thought I was reasonably up-to-date on the topic. However, I did suggest that she talk to her private physician about these things now that she had a little more information. I also gave her some websites to look at if she wanted to search for more information on her own. I was always available if she needed someone to talk with.

Carol thanked me and I left toward my truck to put away my golf equipment.

Perhaps eight years later I was in the snack shop of the golf course getting a drink after I had played the first nine holes. A middle-aged to elderly woman came in about the same time, looked at me, and asked, “Doctor Jimmie, do you remember me?”

I had to confess to the woman that I did not.

She said, “My name is Carol, and you talked to me in the parking lot many years ago about my breast cancer.”

Now I recalled the episode. I said something like, “It appears that you are doing well.”

Carol continued, “I saw my doctor the next day after we talked, and he told me just about everything you told me. In fact, you gave me more information than him. I did not have chemotherapy, but I did have radiation treatments for a short time. I feel great now. I have to tell you that you really relieved my mind that day." She then gave me a hug, kissed my cheek, and walked out to play golf.

The lady who worked behind the counter in the concession area exclaimed, "Doc, looks like you've got a new girlfriend!"

I just picked up my soda and walked to the 10th tee box. I'm sure I had a smile on my face.

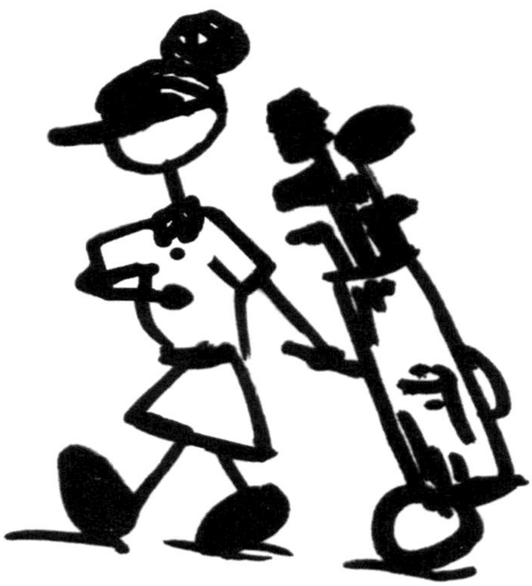

Match Play

I had been playing with the senior golf league for several years before Earl, the coordinator of the match play tournament, kept sweet-talking me to play in the tournament. I knew nothing about match play golf; I did not know the rules or the format, but Earl said it was all for fun. Besides he was the event coordinator, and I didn't want to let him down. Enough arm twisting already. I agreed to play.

A few days before the event, all the players signed in, picked their playing opponent out of a plastic bucket, and received the tournament bracket. The entire tournament was to be played with four-man groups with each pair playing against each other. The tournament was also based on the golf handicap system to make things 'even.' I would come to learn that the handicap system is not perfect.

In match play, you either win or lose a hole. It does not matter what your absolute score is. With the handicap system, to win a hole a golfer's net score just has to be one stroke better than his opponent's net score. Consequently, I learned that if I shot a 4 on a par 4 and my opponent took 10 strokes on a par 4, then I just received credit for winning one hole. Such was the scoring of match play.

With my first opponent, I learned that I had to give him 11 strokes by the handicap system before we even started. A daunting task for sure if I were to win the game. Unfortunately, in this match, I did not play terribly well. Fortunately for me, my opponent played worse than I did. I won by a score of +4 with three holes to play. My opponent headed to the clubhouse to have a beer to drown his sorrows. I continued to play the final three holes on the golf course by myself.

The next day my opponent was Earl himself. Apparently, he had won his first match in a nail-biter on the 18th hole. On this day Earl was having considerable difficulty breathing for reasons unknown to me. Anyway, he was prepared to play the game to keep the tournament on schedule. I found out that I had to give Earl 12 strokes by the handicap system.

As we loaded our clubs onto our golf cart, Earl placed an oxygen cannula on his nose. The cannula was connected to a small oxygen tank in the basket on the rear of the golf cart.

I asked Earl if he was okay to play.

Always joking, Earl said something like, “Fit as a fiddle. Let's do it. Let's have some fun.”

When the other competing twosome was ready to go, we teed off. Earl was first and hit a shot straight down the middle of the fairway. I followed with another shot that landed on the fairway. We were off.

Earl used his oxygen whenever he was in the golf cart for the duration of the match. He briefly removed the nasal cannula only when he was hitting the ball.

After six holes Earl and I were even. However, he won the next three holes so that when we went to the 10th tee box, he was three strokes ahead of me.

One of the fellows playing in the other competing pair was having a dreadful day. By the end of nine holes he was already behind six shots with only nine holes to play.

This team would drop out after a few more holes when one player was down seven shots with only five holes to play.

During the second nine holes I made up a little ground on Earl because I think he was getting tired. However, when we reached the difficult par 3 17th hole,

Earl was still one stroke ahead of me with just two holes to play. Earl would have to score a bogey 4 while I would need to shoot a birdie 2 to win the hole and continue the match.

Earl put his tee shot short of the green. My tee shot landed on the green about 25 feet downhill from the flagstick. I figured my day was over because Earl had been playing very well around the green. I was aware that I had to get a birdie on this hole to keep the match alive.

As I expected, Earl chipped onto the green with his ball stopping within three feet or so from the flagstick. He two-putted for a bogey.

With Earl holding the flagstick, I hit my ball firmly, and it miraculously curved about 2 feet to the left and rolled directly into the cup for a birdie 2. I won the hole; we were tied!

As I was taking the honor by hitting first on our 18th and last hole, Earl was sitting in the golf cart and called out, "Jim, this will be my last hole. I'm all in. I'm all out of air."

I replied, "Earl, you have been short of air all day."

Earl then responded, "I mean I am really out of air!" He showed me the gauge on his oxygen tank which read "0." Earl exclaimed, "See, I REALLY am out of air." He laughed.

I started to laugh. We laughed together.

All I had to do on this hole was to get a par, and I could win the match. However, I was still laughing when I walked to the tee box. Even though I had hit every fairway during the day so far, this tee shot sliced severely to the right and went into the lake. All I could do was chuckle because I was still thinking more about Earl's lack of air comment instead of concentrating on making a good golf shot.

Earl landed his next shot onto the fairway perhaps 150 yards away. That was good enough for me. I conceded the hole and the match and told Earl to go get some oxygen before he croaked on me. Together we chuckled all the way to the clubhouse.

I did not win, but what a way to lose to a nice guy. The match was competitive and, with Earl as my adversary, the game was fun like he said it was supposed to be.

A good lesson for the day.

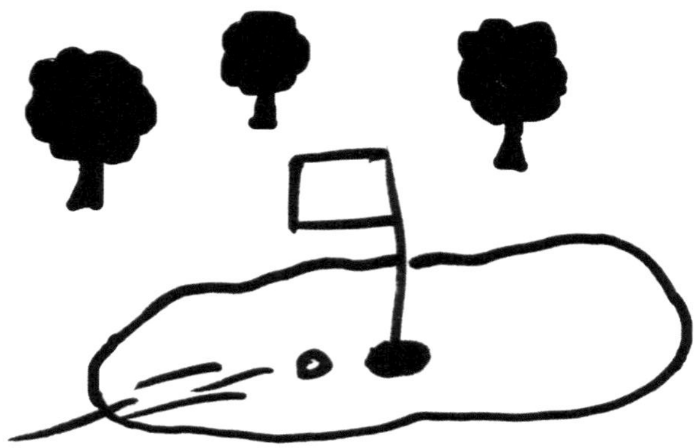

The Complainer

There are some golfers that I call "Poops." These are the golfers who complain about almost everything. They may realize it or not, but they are terribly obnoxious and distracting to their fellow competitors and teammates. A case in point is a golfer named Darwin who I met at an out-of-town golf course. I was part of a team that was playing a two-man best-ball tournament. Once our foursome greeted each other on the first tee box, Darwin immediately told us that he had a lot of trouble hearing, could see like an eagle so we should not lose any of our golf shots, and was very particular about the rules. These comments put the rest of us a bit on edge, but at least, I thought, he was setting his ground rules.

As Darwin was about to make his first tee shot, he asked one of our group to step back from being even with his golf ball because he could see him in his peripheral vision. The golfer moved a bit backward to a point where he thought he was out of Darwin's line of sight. WRONG! Darwin turned to his right and sternly asked the man to move back even farther because the golfer was still standing in his peripheral vision, AND he was moving too much. The golfer stepped back another five steps to be sure that Darwin could not possibly see him.

As Darwin was lining up to hit his ball, he asked one of the other members of our foursome to stop making so much noise chewing his gum! I thought to myself, "This is the guy who said he had trouble hearing?" Darwin finally made a tee shot. The rest of us made our tee shots without nearly as much hullabaloo.

As we were walking toward the fairway, Darwin approached me and told me I was making too much noise with my clubs while he was hitting. At the time of the alleged incident, I was across the tee box and standing still behind him. My clubs were idle in my gold cart. I thought to myself, "So much for being hard of hearing."

Three of our golf balls were in the fairway. Darwin's ball landed a little bit to the left off the fairway. Trying to be a good partner, I gave Darwin his situation as I saw it. He said, "I do not like to hear negative vibes."

Nevertheless, I told Darwin the obvious. His ball was 6 feet behind a tree, he had an out-of-bounds 10 yards to the left, and he had a 120-yard shot to the green. I suggested to him that he consider hitting his ball into the middle of the fairway and take an easy shot onto the green since we were playing as a team.

Darwin repeated, "I don't want to hear any negative thoughts." He then tried to hit his ball through the tree, which obviously failed. The ball got stuck in the tree. Darwin had to take a penalty stroke for an unplayable lie, and he had to drop the ball behind the same tree. Darwin said, "I don't want to hear any more negative vibes."

Darwin ended up scoring a snowman, a score of 8, on the par 4 hole. Fortunately, the remainder of our foursome hit good shots, and we came away with a net birdie on the hole.

On the next hole, Darwin sliced his ball into the right rough. He complained that the tee box ground was uneven causing him to lower his right shoulder. He blamed the uneven ground for his club hitting behind the ball and producing a huge divot in the tee box. This caused him to slice the ball severely. When he hit his next shot out of the rough, the ball soared high into the air and banked severely to the left. Darwin said the grass was too thick. We all saw his ball in the rough. It was positioned on a perfectly flat area of *short* grass.

Darwin's third shot on this hole landed in deep grass next to the green.

Before anyone spoke a word, Darwin said, "I don't want to hear any bad vibes." The rest of us did not whisper a word. Darwin shanked his shot to the right, missed the green entirely, and ended up taking a 7 on a par 4. Thank goodness the rest of our team was able to par the hole.

After two holes of listening to Darwin, the remaining three members of our team did not say another word to him. I for one thought the man had enough troubles of his own between his ears causing his own "bad vibes."

Our foursome managed to get through 18 holes without strangling Darwin. On the 18th hole, Darwin made a putt of at least 40 feet that curved about 2 feet before it rimmed the cup and fell in the hole for a birdie, his first birdie of the day. I went over to congratulate him and said, "Good job, Darwin. It's okay for you to smile now."

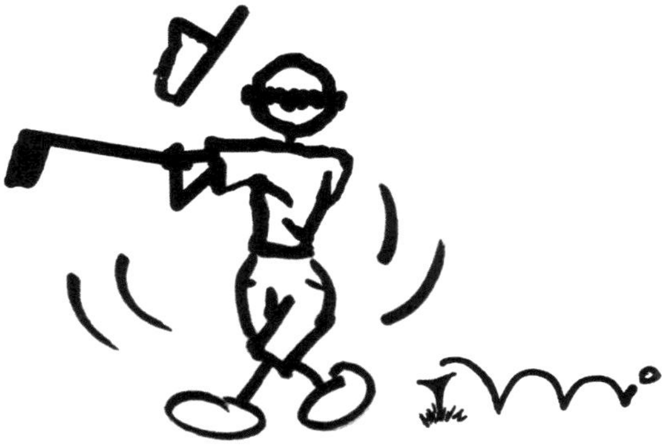

Without smiling his response was, “The ball could've gone straight into the middle of the cup.”

What could I say?

As I entered the clubhouse to hand in our scores, one of the tournament organizers came up to me and asked me how our day went with Darwin. He told me during the last tournament Darwin almost came to blows with one of his partners because of his behavior.

All I could say was, “He is who he is. He's a miserable man, and he's a poop.”

Despite Darwin’s behavior, the rest of our team made quite a few good shots, no one got injured, and our team took second place. All things considered, we had a good day with many lessons.

Vertigo

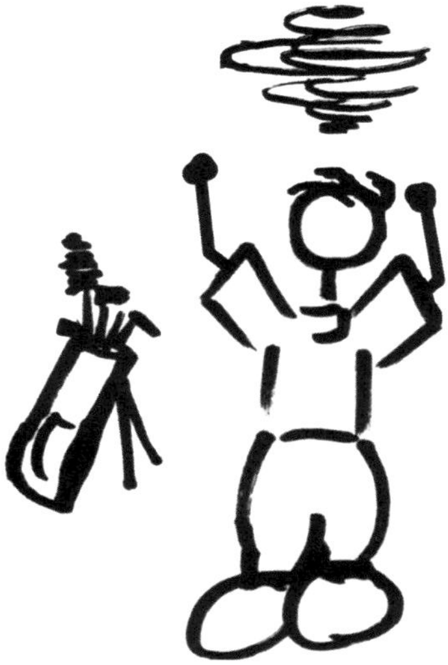

One particular Monday our group started playing our senior league tournament on hole number 8, a 340-yard par 4 hole with a wide straight fairway. Near the landing zone on both sides of the fairway were a few trees and small mounds. An errant shot to the right side would still land on an area with flat ground and short grass; this made an easy shot to the green. The left side of the fairway had deep grass and could cause the golfer some grief. This hole was rated as the easiest one on the golf course.

Doug was one of the golfers in our group. As we were introducing ourselves to each other, Doug made it known that he suffered from vertigo, and sometimes his vertigo caused him to make a bad shot. At the same time that Doug was talking to us, he was touching his toes, twisting his body, moving his head from left to right, and then practicing his swing with a long follow through.

I thought to myself, “There is no way this fellow has vertigo.”

Vertigo is a sensation of whirling and loss of balance, associated particularly with looking down or moving the head. It can be caused by a disease affecting the inner ear and the body’s balance mechanism. Often the person is nauseous and has to sit or lie down until the symptoms resolve.

Having cared for many patients over the years with vertigo symptoms, I knew this man had none of them. Anyway, I just let him talk and didn't say a word.

Doug's first drive of the day was not very good. The ball sliced severely to the right, and I do mean severely. It landed on another fairway. Doug promptly shook his head side to side and said, “Damn vertigo!” Then he said, “Hey men, pardon my French.” I just knew this guy was going to be a handful for our group.

Doug's ball made it to the green after three more shots. As he was getting ready to putt, Doug paced back and forth around the green looking at the potential path of his ball. All the while I could not help but notice that he was walking with a steady gait with his head moving back-and-forth and up-and-down without any signs of dizziness. Finally, Doug made a putt that was several feet off-line. He said, “There’s that vertigo again.” Without further theatrics, Doug tapped his put in for a triple bogey seven.

Hole number 9, a par 4 that is rated as the most difficult hole on the outward side of the golf course, was our next challenge. After three of us hit our tee shots,

Doug hammered a drive about 220 yards down the center of the fairway. Doug said, "Thank goodness, no vertigo that time."

The remaining three members of our group just looked at each other and wondered, "What gives with this guy?"

One of the golfers quietly asked me, "Doc, can dizziness come and go just like that?"

I replied, "No way."

Doug's second shot to the 9th green was about 150 yards. He shanked this shot about 45° to the right into the adjoining lake. We all heard Doug exclaim, "There goes that damn vertigo again!" Eventually, Doug's ball made it to the green. He finally putted 4 times to score an 8, a snowman.

Doug's shenanigans continued for the remainder of our game. When he had a good shot, he had no vertigo, and Doug made sure we knew that his vertigo had vanished for that good shot. However, whenever he had a bad shot, and there were many, Doug placed the blame on his chronic vertigo.

A par score for the nine holes that we played was 36. Doug scored 60. I calculated that he suffered about 48 episodes of "vertigo" in a timeframe of about two hours. I surmised that if Doug really did have intermittent chronic vertigo the way he presented itself this day, then he should be studied at a medical center. Otherwise, I figured he had some type of mental dysfunction, or he just needed to have a reason for his lack of golfing talent. Anyway, his behavior was annoying and a distraction, and, at the end of the day, comical, at least to me.

One member of our group told me that Doug suffered from the golfing disease of too much LOFT.

I asked him what was LOFT?

He whispered in my ear, “Lack Of Freaking Talent.”

I nodded in agreement without saying a word.

I saw Doug in the parking lot putting away his golf equipment into the trunk of his car. In the process, I saw him bending over up-and-down and twisting his head left and right without any sign whatsoever of wanting to fall over.

As I passed by him, I wished Doug the best for the rest of the day. I told him that I hoped his “vertigo" would get better as the day went on.

Doug said, “I'm feeling pretty good now. I think I'm going to have a good day.”

Yet another golf lesson for me today.

The Number 5

Usually, a foursome has one player who acts as a scorekeeper for the team. This becomes particularly important during events, such as our senior league tournaments, when cumulative scores of all the players are important for final team scores and personal handicap ratings. I, for one, have always kept my own scorecard when I play just so I can compare my scores with our team's official scorecard. Many golfers, but not all, keep their own scorecards. Some golfers rely solely on the honesty, reliability, and integrity of the official scorekeeper.

Our senior league has arrangements with multiple other golf courses in our area to supply a four-man team to play in what's called inter-club tournaments during the summer. I was chosen to be part of one of these inter-club teams one year. I had the opportunity to play golf at one of the private golf courses in our town for the first time.

I made sure that I arrived at the course early so I could learn about any local rules that may affect the golf game. The club's golf professional gave me the names of the players on my team and the golf clubs they represented. Forty golfers were participating that day representing ten golf clubs.

All of the golfers gathered in the pro shop for our final instructions for the 2-net-best-ball tournament, and a member of each foursome was given the official scorecard. As the members of my foursome met each other and introduced ourselves, we chose one member from the host course named Frank to be our team's scorekeeper. The man had been a member of the course for many years and told us that he was "a real numbers man." Apparently, Frank had been an accountant, an actuary, and on the executive finance team at a regional bank for many years. He said he had recently retired at the age of 70. Without hesitation, we gave Frank the scorekeeping responsibility for the team.

The first hole was a par 4. Three of our team parred the hole and one got a bogey. However, adding in our individual handicaps, our net score was one under par.

The second hole was a par 5. Our team scored two 5s and two 6s. With our handicaps, however, our net score was 2 more strokes under par.

The third hole was a par 3. Our scores included a birdie 2, two par 3s, and a five. Our handicaps netted us another 2 strokes under par.

One of the guys asked Frank how we were doing.

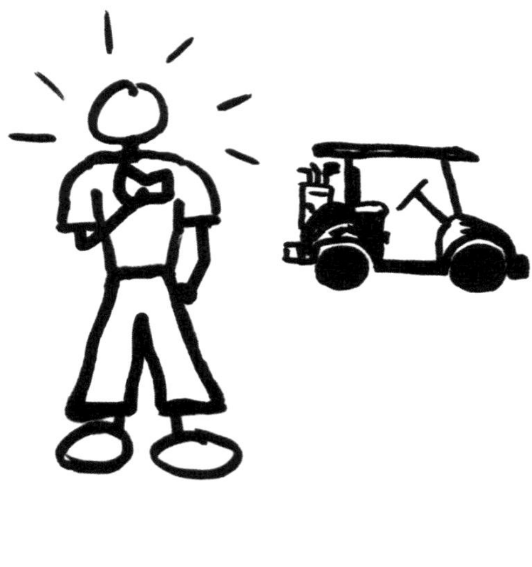

Frank replied, “It doesn't look like we're doing too well yet men. We're going to have to step it up if we think we're going to win this tournament.”

One player asked Frank, “What do you mean? We should be about five under par after only three holes.” With that comment, the golfer asked Frank to show him the scorecard. The man then exclaimed, “What the heck?”

Frank asked if there was a problem.

The golfer said something like, “Well heck yeah! All you've written down are 5s for each of us on each hole. You have our team score well over par. You didn’t figure in our handicaps either. We should be 5 under par.”

Frank then told us that since his stroke a few months before he had been having a little trouble concentrating.

It appeared that no matter what score we gave Frank, he just entered 5s for everyone for whatever reason.

Since I was riding with Frank in the same golf cart, I offered to take over the scoring duties for the team. However, I asked each of the other members to keep their own scores so that we could compare them when we were finished. I wanted to make sure I didn't make any more errors.

They agreed.

I did not have a pencil with an eraser to correct our scorecard nor did any the other members of our team. However, Frank suggested using the end of a golf grip as an eraser. I did not know this trick, but it worked pretty well.

After I erased and corrected the score card to everyone's satisfaction, we continued to play. I think Frank apologized to me on every hole. He kept telling me it was hell to get old.

Our team played and scored well; we ended up in second place. We each received $40 in pro shop credit.

At the end, Frank was most courteous to his teammates and said he appreciated the fact that we didn't make too much out of his scorekeeping snafu. He thought that his scorekeeping days were done.

I told Frank that he did not have to keep score to have fun playing golf.

Another good lesson for me.

Play The Ball Where It Lies

With a shotgun start our foursome started on the 8th hole. Our golf round was going pretty well for three of the four members of our group. Josh, however, was having one of those difficult golfing days. I do not believe that his golf ball landed on a single fairway for our first seven holes. His shots were slicing to the right, they were hooking to the left, and they were bouncing every which way except onto the fairways. He even managed to lose two golf balls in the water. Despite his misfortunes, Josh remained positive that he could do better.

Our group eventually reached the 6th hole, which has a 45° dogleg turn to the right. The turn in the fairway is protected by several evergreen trees. One member of our foursome suggested to Josh that he consider aiming a little bit left to see if he could finally get a ball to land on the fairway. I could not tell from my vantage point how Josh addressed his ball or where he was aiming. However, he managed to hit a drive high into the air that sliced severely toward the lake on the right side of the tee box and a good forty yards from the fairway.

Guarding the lake from errant golf shots were several large cottonwood trees. We all saw Josh's ball hit the first big tree. Usually, when this occurs the ball falls into the lake. However, none of us saw where the ball came to rest, nor did we see a splash of water from the lake.

Since our team had three balls in the fairway awaiting our second shots, we went as a group looking for Josh's golf ball. Amazingly, the ball had dropped straight down on the fairway side of the tree which gave Josh an opportunity for a good second shot back toward the fairway.

Instead of chipping his ball sideways back onto the fairway, Josh decided he could cut the corner of the dogleg with his second shot. All he had to do was hit a shot high enough to get over the evergreen trees. He failed! The second shot landed about 6 feet up into one of the evergreen trees.

After the remainder of our foursome had hit their second shots toward the green, we went over to survey Josh's predicament.

We all saw the ball on a branch of the evergreen tree a few inches from the end of a branch and at Josh's eye level. One of our group suggested to Josh that he take an unplayable lie and drop the ball beside the tree where he would have an open shot to the green.

Josh was convinced he could hit his ball out of the tree. We all stepped back to watch him hit his ball.

Josh took out his driver, I assumed because it had the biggest head, and took a mighty baseball-like swing. With his first attempt he missed the tree entirely, a whiff. Josh was encouraged again to take an unplayable lie and just drop his ball. He told us, "The rule book says to play the ball where it lies. So that's what I'm going to do."

With his next swing, Josh hit the tree branch which only knocked his ball farther toward the center of the tree. After this failed attempt, one frustrated member of our foursome finally went up to Josh, pointed to his driver in his hand, and said, "Josh, now think about this. You have a used golf ball in the tree worth maybe a quarter. You are trying to ruin a four-hundred-dollar driver just so you can hit a twenty-five-cent golf ball. Take the unplayable lie penalty and hit the freaking ball off the ground!"

After this exchange we started to laugh. Even Josh chuckled. Josh left his ball in the tree, took his unplayable lie penalty, dropped another ball, and hit it not even close to the green into more deep-grass rough and more trouble. Josh finished the hole with a well-earned score of 10.

On our last hole of the day Josh hit what I call a P O (pissed off) shot. His last drive of the day went straight and true down the middle of the fairway about 230 yards.

What could we say? We cheered for him. Josh ended his golf day with at least one good shot.

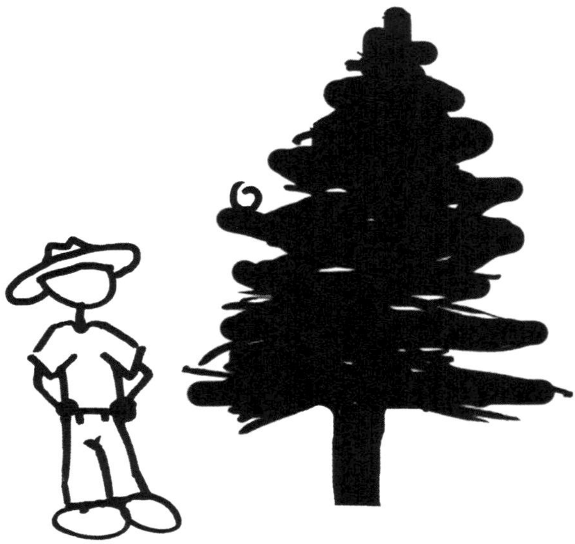

"Experience is not what happens to you. It is what you do with what happens to you."

Aldous Huxley

The Sandbagger

The game for the day was a scramble. The simple rules of a scramble are (1) each golfer hits from the tee box and the best shot is chosen, (2) the same process occurs with each successive shot until the ball goes into the cup, (3) and each golfer is required to use his or her tee shot at least once every nine holes.

On the first tee box three of our foursome hit their balls onto the fairway. Freddie, our fourth player and the highest handicap player in our group, hit his ball from the forward tees used by the high handicap players. The ball struck the end of his 1-wood and soared 90° to the right into the rough. We didn't even spend the time looking for the ball because it was so far into the deep grass, and we would not use his drive on this hole anyhow. Collectively, our foursome made our way down the fairway with three of us walking and Freddie driving his cart.

After we chose what we collectively decided was the best drive of the three remaining balls on the fairway, each of us in sequence hit a second shot. Freddie yanked his shot severely to the left out of bounds into a lake. Fortunately, one of our other shots landed on the green close to the flagstick so that our team was able to putt for a potential birdie.

Freddie putted first to give the rest of us a good line on where the putt was going to go. He hit the ball entirely too hard and crooked. The ball stopped about 2 feet off-line and 10 feet past the hole. Freddie apologized for not being terribly helpful. As luck would have it, the next player made a nice putt for a birdie.

The next seven holes became a replay of the very first hole with regard to Freddie's inability to strike the golf ball. He lost about six ball. Along the way, however, our team managed to score 4 more birdies so that by the time we reached our 9th hole of the day our team score was 5 shots under par. Unfortunately, our team had not yet used Freddie's drive. I for one was doubtful about where his ball would end up on the golf course after his tee shot.

After three of us hit our shots from the regular tee box, Freddie drove his cart to the forward tee area and took his position to hit. Just as we walked up to Freddie's cart, he stroked his drive. Unbelievably, the ball went straight down the fairway coming to rest near the 100-yard marker located in the center of the fairway. The ball was only about 95 yards from the flagstick. Freddie promptly hopped into his golf cart and sped away down the fairway toward his ball.

We remaining three golfers started walking down the fairway in total amazement at Freddie’s excellent shot.

When we were about 30 yards from Freddie's ball in the middle of the fairway, we saw Freddie get out of his golf cart, take aim, and hit a low screaming shot toward the green. We all saw that the ball landed in front of the green, made a few small bounces, and finally came to rest a short distance from the flagstick. We spontaneously let out a big hoot congratulating Freddie on his second consecutive magnificent shot.

Before we could reach Freddie and congratulate him, he was back in his golf cart speeding toward the green. He parked his golf cart on the cart path on the far side of the green. After choosing his putter, Freddie confidently strolled to his ball and tapped it in for a birdie 3. He then sauntered back to his cart, sat behind the steering wheel with his arms crossed, and waited for the three of us to make our way to the green. Freddie had not hit a good shot all day. Now he stroked three successive shots with precision and scored a point for our team all by himself!

When we arrived at Freddie's cart, one of the fellows told Freddie, “You are such a sandbagger! Fantastic job!” We then embarrassed Freddie with a group hug.

We were all pretty happy for Freddie. His birdie on that 9th hole put our team at 6 under par and our team took first place for that day’s event.

We had an amazing day! What a lesson!

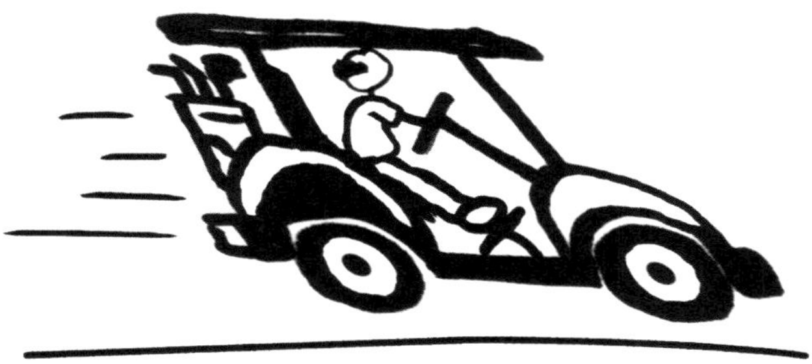

"You guys are playing slower than my mother,
and she's dead!"
Anonymous

Optimism

Hole number 15 which is a par 4 about 370 yards with a 45° dogleg deviation to the right was the starting hole for our group this Monday morning. The bend in the dogleg is protected by a group of trees and mounds. A lake borders most of the left side of the fairway.

One member of our foursome on this particular day was a fellow named Raymond. He was a hunched-over frail appearing fellow who was in his mid-80s I guessed. I had played with him once before. I knew he was a Korean War veteran because his hat said so. Raymond was our high handicap player for the day. After three of our group made their tee shots, Raymond walked to the forward tee box which was reserved for high handicap players and those players over 80 years.

Raymond lined up to hit his ball straight down the middle of the fairway, he took a robust swing for him, and his golf ball careened about 45° to his left. The ball bounced several times before it went into the lake. Raymond just stood there on the tee box with his right arm propped up by his golf club and stared at the water. He said something like, "Now how did I do that?"

He then started to walk the short distance toward the place where his ball entered the water. He called out that he was taking the penalty stroke, and he would be shooting 3.

Raymond's partner in the golf cart pulled up beside him. Raymond pulled out a different golf club, and took another mighty swing. This time his club hit the ground behind the golf ball taking out a substantial divot of sod, and the ball bounced slowly to his left before trickling into the lake again. Raymond's response was something like, "Well I'll be jiggered! Did you see that? I can't believe it."

He then started walking toward the location where we, as a group, concluded that his ball went into the water. We searched briefly in the lake for his ball, but the water was too murky for us to see much except for the catfish coming to the surface to catch a meal.

Raymond dropped another ball. He stated, "In the water in 3, out in 4, hitting 5." He lined up to take his fifth shot on this par 4 hole. With this swing his back foot slipped on some wet grass, and his ball bolted straight into the lake. Raymond apologized to us and said, "I can't believe I'm hitting the ball like this today. I'm usually not this bad guys."

Raymond took out yet another golf ball, dropped it on to the ground after measuring two club lengths from the lake's edge, and pronounced loudly, "In the lake in 5, out in 6, hitting 7. Let's just hope I hit this one a little bit better."

Raymond's ball was now lying about 100 yards away from the flagstick. He took another vigorous swing; the ball took off nicely and bounced several times before it approached the green with the flagstick about thirty feet from the edge of the green. The ball rolled smoothly right into the middle of the hole for a score of 7.

The rest of us let out a hoot. When our group gathered on the green, Raymond said with a big grin, "Did you guys see that? I got a hole-in-one! This is going to be a good golf day. I can feel it."

As we were making our way to the next tee box, I mentioned to Raymond then he had some pretty bad luck on the last hole.

Raymond looked me in the eye and replied, "Young man, the North Koreans could not kill me. The Chinese could not kill me. An artillery bombardment at 20 below zero could not kill me. I just don't believe that hitting a golf ball into the water is going to do me much damage." He then said, "I just feel like I'm going to have a good day today."

For the next eight holes, Raymond became our star player. Since he was our team's highest handicap player, he got the most bonus shots, and he gave our team a lot of those bonus shots. Our team managed to score well enough to take first place and earn those all-important pro shop credits.

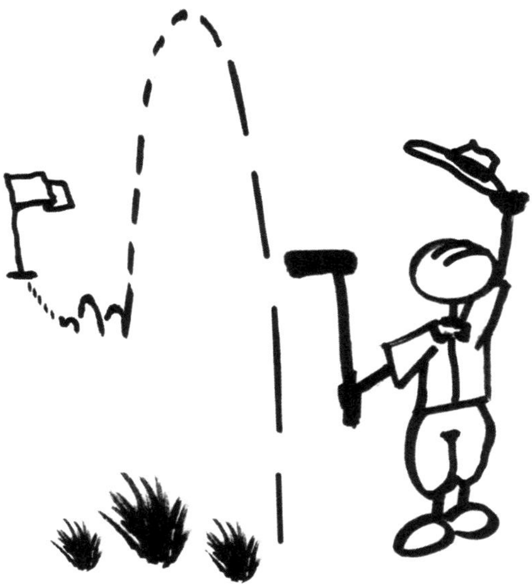

"If I hit it right, it's sliced. If I hit it left, it's a hook.
If I hit it straight, it's a miracle."
Anonymous

Bionic Septuagenarians

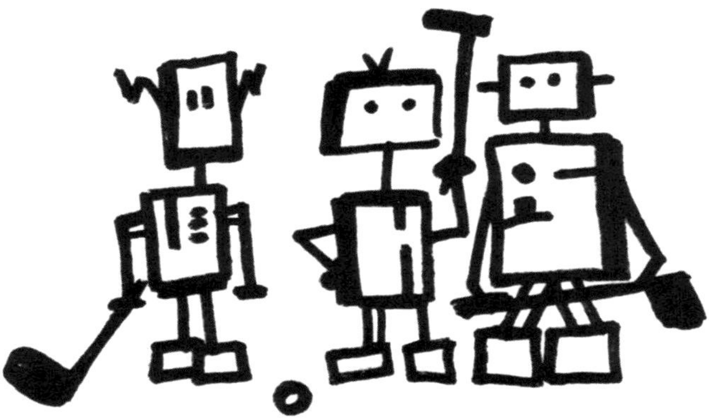

The lady in the golf shop directed me to the 10th tee area to join up with three gentleman who were about ready to play. She then called to them on the loudspeaker to make sure they waited for me. Upon my arrival at the tee box each of the men who appeared to be in their 70s greeted me cordially.

The first man said his name was Maurice, or better known to his friends as "Moe." The second man shook my hand and said, "My name is Lawrence but most people call me Larry." The final golfer grabbed my hand to shake it with both of his hands. He said his name was Cedric.

He then removed his hat to reveal a totally bald head. With a big grin and a laugh, he said, "Just call me Curly, my friends do."

As we sauntered down the first fairway looking for our golf balls after our tee shots, it became obvious to me that these three fellows were good friends. In fact, one of them told me that they had gone to school together in a small town outside of Billings and were affectionately known in high school as Moe, Larry, and Curly, the Three Stooges.

I smiled and had a good chuckle.

On the next tee box I noticed that Moe had vertical scars on the front of both his knees. After he had completed his golf shot, I mentioned to him that I had noticed his leg scars. Moe told me that he had both knees replaced the previous fall and winter. Before that he had both hips replaced. He laughed and quipped that he couldn't go through a scanner at the airport any longer without setting off all the alarms.

It was at this time that Moe asked me what I did for living when I worked. When I told him that I was a physician in a small town in Montana for many years and then a medical educator, Moe said I might be interested in the trio for their medical issues. I just listened and didn't reply.

Larry overheard what Moe and I had been saying on the tee box. Laughingly, he pronounced that not only were the three of them called the Three Stooges but also they had been named the bionic trio because over the years they had pretty much been put back together by doctors with the advances in medicine. Larry then pointed out that he had had his neck fused the year before with titanium plates and screws. Prior to that he underwent two surgeries on his low back and a hip replacement.

Curly had driven nearby with his golf cart. Overhearing part of our conversations and wanting to put in his two cents worth, he told me that he was using a golf cart because his doctor didn't want him to walk too much for a month. Apparently, his hip was replaced just 10 days before and Curly was still undergoing rehabilitation for the surgery. Curly also informed me that he had one total knee replacement, a shoulder replacement, and he was looking forward to his other hip being replaced at the end of the golf season.

I thought to myself, "I am playing with three bionic septuagenarians, AND they're all playing better than me!" I was truly impressed.

As we continued with our golf game I learned that all three gentlemen were widowers. Not only were they best buddies throughout their school years but now that they were all in their late 70s the trio had become their own small support group.

As we were finishing up our golf round on the 18th green, with a big grin on my face and to keep myself from laughing, I shook the hands of Moe, Larry, and Curly in sequence and thanked them for their lessons.

"How well did I play? Today I played with my one-year-old great grandson. He won!"

Anonymous

Birth Defects

One of the necessities of playing golf is to have a clean golf ball. There are multiple ways to keep your golf ball clean. Some of these include wiping the ball with a wet towel, placing the ball in a specifically designed handheld accessory just for cleaning, spitting on the ball, wiping the ball with your hands or clothing, licking the ball, licking a part of your hand and then rubbing the ball, or various combinations of any of the above.

One morning during a senior golf event our foursome met one of the groundskeepers who was applying a chemical to the green. When asked, the gentleman told us that he was attempting to kill a certain kind of weed and fungus on the greens. We wished him good luck; we complimented him on the work he and the groundskeepers did to make the course nice.

On the next hole my approach shot sailed high into the air and made a substantial divot in the green when it landed. After repairing my ball mark and after marking my ball placement, I licked my thumb to clean off my ball. One member of our foursome pointed out to me that the chemicals being applied to the greens that morning could cause me to have birth defects. With sincerity, he admonished the other members of our foursome not to clean their ball by licking them, licking their fingers and cleaning them, or in any way becoming in contact with the chemicals being applied to the green. Again, he noted that the chemicals caused birth defects.

One of the members of our foursome asked him exactly what kind of birth defects could we experience since we were already in our 60s or 70s.

Looking the golfer directly in the eyes he said, "You could be born without an arm or leg or have something else missing. You could even be born retarded."

The remaining three golfers in our foursome looked at each other, smiled, and rolled our eyes upward. I thought to myself, "What is he talking about!"

To satisfy this gentleman, however, we made sure that we cleaned our golf balls only with a towel for the rest of the morning. Afterward, we were all "relieved" that we were not born again with a missing arm or leg or something worse.

Three Georges

It was my third week of senior league golf when I was 61 years old. Our foursome started off on hole #1. Before we started the game, the members of foursome introduced themselves to each other. Frequently, and most often in my experience, the golfers may give just their first names. On this occasion, I introduced myself to my first teammate who was a powerfully built man in his 70s. He told me to call him George.

I introduced myself to the second golfer who appeared to be a bit older. He said, "My name is George." So now I had George the big and George the small. I wrote this on my scorecard so I would remember who I was talking to.

I introduced myself to the third golfer on my team.

While sporting a big grin, he said, "My name is George. Just call me George."

Now I had George #1, George #2, and George #3 written on my scorecard so I could remember their names. I told the man that I was old and confused, so I asked them what their full names were. They replied in sequence George Alston, George Herbert, and George Larson.

I just knew that Earl, who arranged the foursomes for senior league play that year, had set me up with three men named George just for fun.

As we started to play, I could see and feel that these players were way out of my league. They hit the ball straight and true, and I hit the ball long and crooked. They had a good touch around the greens, and it was obvious that I did not have a clue how to hit a good shot around the greens. They putted like professionals, and I felt like a hack. By the third hole, I was thoroughly demoralized, psyched out, and overwhelmed playing with these quality players.

On our 4th hole, I yanked my ball just off the fairway into the rough on the left side. After I miss hit my second shot and still in the rough, I pulled out what I thought would be an appropriate club when George Herbert came up beside me and said, “Why don't you try using your seven iron. Place the ball by your back foot, swing down on the ball not so hard, and allow the ball to roll onto the green.”

I thought to myself, “What the heck. I'll give it a try.”

Hallelujah! The ball did just as George Herbert said it would. I thanked him for his tip.

On the next hole, my tee shot went through the fairway and landed in grass about 3 inches tall. I was only about 100 yards away. George Alston came up to me and asked me what I was going to do. I told him at 100 yards, I should be able to get to the green with a sand wedge. George Alston suggested that because of the deep grass I might consider using one club higher, a pitching wedge. Since a strong wind was directly into our faces, he suggested that I add an additional club to compensate for the wind which made my club choice now a nine iron. I thought his comments were logical. And, what the heck, I was just learning how to play the game anyway.

Instead of using a sand wedge for a 100-yard shot, I used a 9 iron, two clubs higher. I hit my ball squarely and it came out of the heavy grass quite nicely. It bounced once before it slowly rolled onto the green. After seeing the results of my shot, I thanked George Alston for his help.

The other three players in my foursome obviously were more accomplished at playing golf then I. I was definitely a newbie, in awe, and my play proved it.

As we were about to tee off on our ninth and final hole, George Larson, George #3, said, "Why don't we tell this young man who we are?" They all grinned as they told me of their golfing achievements. Each had been an accomplished golfer for over 40 years. Collectively, the trio recounted the number of country club championships, Montana State amateur championships, and senior championships they had won. I felt that I was in a group of senior golfing royalty since I had been golfing seriously for only about a year. I thanked them all for the lessons.

When we handed in our scorecard in the clubhouse, Earl was at the scorer's table. He had a big smile on his face, and he appeared to be waiting for me. He said, "Hey Jim, did you have a good day?"

I smiled, told Earl that I learned a lot, and thanked him for taking good care of me.

Earl just said, "Jim, you're welcome."

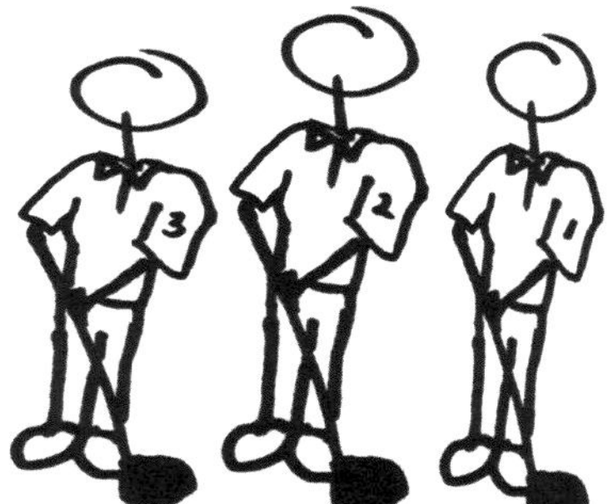

"If I was playing in a two-man scramble,
I would have finished third."
Anonymous

Cystic Fibrosis

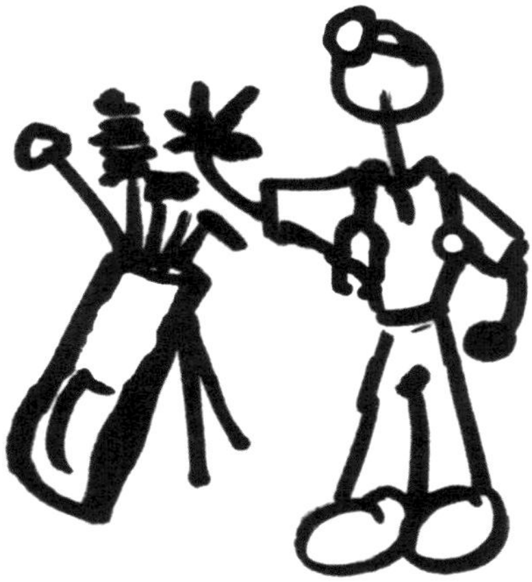

As I was warming up on the driving range one morning before the senior league started, one of the other golfers waved his arm and said something like, "Hey Doc, good morning! I hope you play well and have a good round."

I responded in kind with good wishes.

As I was cleaning one of my irons in the water bucket, yet another golfer came up beside me and said, "I heard someone call you 'Doc'. Are you like a real doctor?"

I introduced myself and told the fellow that I was indeed a real medical doctor. I asked him if he had a question for me.

He told me his name was Harmon, and he wanted to know if I had a minute to answer a question he had.

I had been in this scenario many times before as people were seeking more answers to the medical questions that their private doctors may not have answered completely. I told him that I would be glad to answer his question if I could. However, I also informed Harmon that I was no longer a practicing clinical physician. I did tell him, however, that I had a wealth of experience in a multitude of areas of medicine.

When he started to ask a question, I could see tears welling up in his eyes.

Before he could say too much and to give the man some time to compose himself, I asked him how old he was.

He told me he was 77 years old. He then told me that he learned the day before that he had "Cystic Fibrosis" and was going to die! His doctor did not give him any idea of treatment for the disease. Harmon wanted to know if I knew anything about cystic fibrosis.

Being the tactless fellow that I can be at times, I told the fellow bluntly that I knew that he did not have, and absolutely could not have, cystic fibrosis. I informed him that cystic fibrosis is a childhood disease and that children usually do not live more than 15 to 20 years. Since he was now 76 years old, I knew that he could not possibly have cystic fibrosis. I asked Harmon to give me more information.

He told me that he went to the doctor because he was having trouble breathing. He could no longer walk 18 holes for a round of golf without becoming exhausted.

When I asked Harmon if he ever smoked cigarettes, he said, "Well yeah, since I was 16 years old, almost 60 years."

I then asked Harmon what the doctor actually told him.

He said his doctor sent him to the radiologist for some pictures of his chest. Afterward, he spoke with the radiologist about what he saw. Harmon recalled that the radiologist showed him white areas on the pictures that he called fibrosis or scarring in his lungs. The films also revealed small, dark circular areas in his lungs that looked like small balloons. The doctor called them cysts.

I knew right then that Harman had incorrectly interpreted what the doctor had said. What the doctor described, in medical terms, was advanced pulmonary emphysema with fibrosis and bullae, or cysts. Harmon heard only "cystic fibrosis."

I asked Harmon how long he wanted to live.

He told me that never really thought about it.

I suggested to Harmon that he talk with his doctor seriously about his diagnosis, any treatment that was available, and to make sure he had a will.

The next time I saw Harmon at the golf course he was riding in a golf cart. I could see that he was using continuous oxygen, and he gave me two thumbs up as he headed off to the first tee box.

Harmon was able to play golf until his early 80s.

"I know that you believe you understand what you think I said, but I'm not sure you realize that what you heard is not what I meant."
Robert McCloskey

A Miracle

Terry was the high handicap player for our team one Monday morning in senior league play. I had played golf with Terry and his wife once before on a weekend. He did not play golf very well that day. Terry was a year older than me and had played collegiate football in his younger years. He was still a large powerful man, but his days of playing football had taken a significant toll on his joints and flexibility. The first day I played with Terry and his wife, he shot about 65 to 70 for nine holes. His official handicap for nine holes was the maximum of 18 strokes. I didn't think that 18 strokes were nearly enough for Terry's game.

Before we started our game, which was a 2-net-best-ball tournament, I briefly chatted with Terry about how he had been doing. He told me his golf game really sucked. He said that he and his wife played the day before on Sunday, and she beat him by 10 strokes. He continued with, "That should tell you in a nutshell how good my golf game is."

Having played with Terry before, his comment did not surprise me. I only hoped he would have a better day.

We started on the 7th hole which is a straightaway par 5 about 500 yards long. After three of us had hit our tee shots, Terry clobbered his drive straight down the fairway about 250 yards. With a smile, he said, "I wonder where that came from?"

Terry hit his second shot straight down the fairway again. He turned around, looked at me, raised his arms in triumph, and just smiled. I remembered playing with Terry before, and he did not hit two straight shots onto the fairway the entire round.

Terry's third shot on the par five hole wasn't pretty, but the ball bounced its way onto the green. Yahoo! He would be putting for a birdie! He then hit a 25-foot putt that dropped in the hole for a birdie. His high handicap gave our team two strokes. His birdie putt awarded us another stroke. Another member of our team made a birdie also. We received one stroke for his handicap and one stroke for his birdie. Our team scored a net 5 shots under par on the first hole.

The next hole, which was rated the easiest hole on the golf course, was a 339-yard par 4. Terry hit his drive far to the right near the previous fairway where a stand of trees stood between him and the green. His next shot bounced somewhere among the trees and came to rest at the base of one of the trees. Terry had essentially a blind shot to the green. Actually, the rest of us did not see Terry when he hit his third shot. All we heard was a whack before we saw a ball hit on a mound to the right side of the green and then bounce toward the flagstick. The ball hit the flagstick with considerable force, but fell straight down into the hole for a birdie 3.

For the birdie, Terry scored one point for our team. His high handicap gave us another 2 points. Another member of our foursome received another point when he scored a par and received one point for his handicap. For this hole, our team scored an additional net four strokes under par.

Our team's next hole, the 9th, was rated as the most difficult on the front side of the golf course. It was a 390-yard par 4 hole with a slight dogleg to the left. The left side of the fairway was protected by mounds and trees. Most of the right side of the fairway bordered two lakes and a lateral water hazard. Placing the ball in the middle of the fairway was paramount to scoring well.

Having scored a birdie on the previous hole, Terry was given the honors to hit first. The last time I played with Terry on this hole, he sliced his ball well into the lake on the right side. Today, however, Terry hit a screaming line drive down the middle of the fairway about 250 yards. All he could do was spin around from the tee box, shrug his shoulders, and smile.

Terry's second shot was not technically very good. He hit the ground behind his ball producing a monstrous divot. However, his ball had a lot of topspin which made it roll, and roll, and roll until it finally limped onto the green about 120 yards away.

The other two members of our foursome just started to laugh because of the shots that Terry was making. The shots were not pretty, but they were getting the job done. I told Terry not to worry because there were no points for style in golf. Amazingly, Terry putted just once on this hole to score yet another birdie 3. With this birdie and his handicap score, Terry garnered another three points for our team. Another member of our team with a high handicap also scored a par which gave us another net 2 points for our team. All together, we left this hole with an additional 5 shots under par.

Terry continued his amazing shot making for the remainder of the nine-hole tournament, but his scoring cooled off a bit. Our other higher handicap player also continued to score well. Our final scorecard showed that our team had scored 10 points better than the next lowest scoring team. Par was 36 for the nine holes that we played. According to his handicap, Terry should have had a gross score of 54 or more. His final gross score was 40. His net score of 22.

When we handed in our scorecard, the golfers at the scoring table looked incredulous when they saw our score. They were especially dubious about Terry's net score of 22.

I saw the look on their faces and reassured them that I was keeping score, our entire team verified the score, and Terry had the most amazing round of golf in his life. What a difference a day can make, especially for golfers.

At the end of the year when awards were given out, Terry received the "Sandbagger of the Year" award for the lowest net score recorded during the league year. He received a few dollars in prize money and a small bucket of dirt!

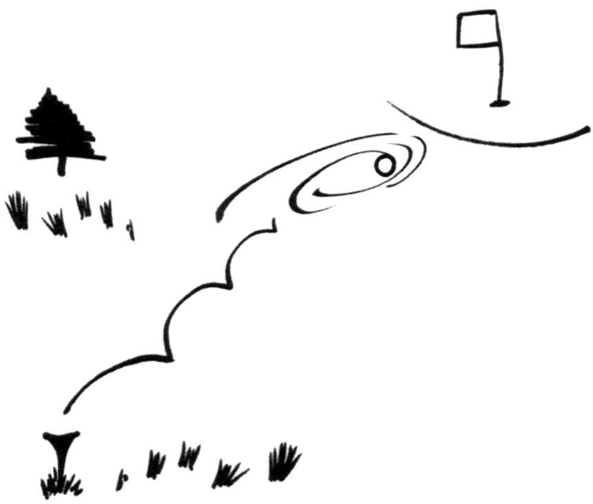

Assisted Hole-in-One

Our foursome for senior league play was about ready to tee off on our second hole this particular morning. Our challenge was the 133-yard par 3 number 13 hole at the Yegen Golf Club in Billings, Montana. To the right of the tee box is a lake. To the left of the tee box is a lateral water hazard (irrigation ditch) that is snuggled closely to an out-of-bounds barbed-wire fence. One of the groundskeepers was mowing the tee box area as we were about ready to hit. As our foursome was waiting for the group on the green to finish the hole, the groundskeeper dismounted his mower and came over to talk to us. He told us that the day before he had scored a hole-in-one on the same hole we were going to play. The man continued to describe how he hit a low screaming line drive that he thought was going to fly over the green and out of bounds. Instead, the ball hit the flagstick and fell directly into the cup. He told us that we could read about his accomplishment in the newspaper the next day.

The members of our group complimented the fellow for his fine shot.

Curtis, a member of our foursome, pronounced, "I scored a hole-in-one on this hole last year"

Jason, another member of our foursome who knew Curtis and also knew that Curtis liked to tell golf stories, said, "Oh yeah."

Curtis replied, "I'm not kidding!"

Jason noted that he had not seen Curtis's name in the paper for getting a hole-in-one.

Curtis responded with, "When I got the hole-in-one I was a little embarrassed." He then continued to tell us that he had not hit the ball well. It hit the sidewalk located just past the edge of the lake and bounced high into the air. Somehow, the ball made its way onto the green. The flagstick was positioned that day just a few steps onto the front of the green. The members of his foursome watched as a goose flew from the lake, waddled onto the green and pecked his ball into the cup for a hole-in-one.

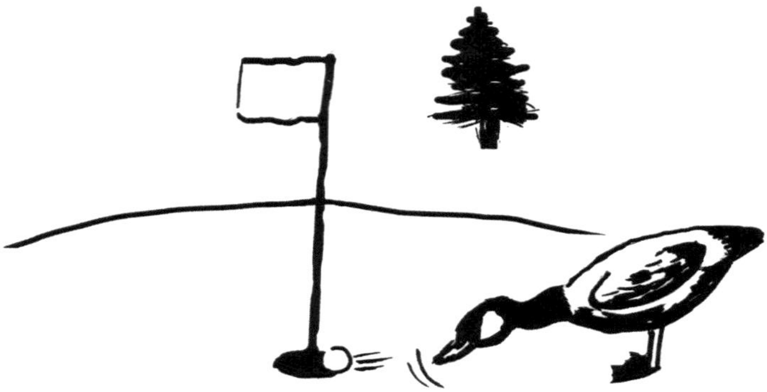

Jason retorted, “Curtis, you are so full of it!”

To this comment Curtis replied that his group was not sure if the shot should count as a hole-in-one. However, after the round they explained the episode to the golf pro.

The golf pro told them that indeed it was counted as a hole-in-one. He explained that the goose was a natural object. The hole-in-one counted just as if the ball had bounced off the sidewalk into the hole, or bounced off a rock or a fence or anything else. As long as one of the golfers did not physically touch the ball after it was hit, the hole-in-one counted.

Jason noted, "That's unbelievable!"

Curtis then called out by name to one of the golfers who were just leaving the green and related that he was explaining his goose assisted hole-in-one.

The golfer yelled back, "One hell of a shot! One for the books for sure. I was there and all four of us saw it happen."

Jason asked Curtis why he didn't record it in the newspaper.

Curtis answered that the goose was the one who should take credit for his lucky "goose-and-one."

"The only thing I didn't hit well today was my golf ball."
Anonymous

A Direct Hit

Sometime in the early years of the twenty-first century the city and the golf club came to an agreement that allowed an easement on golf club property for the construction of a city street with the purpose of improving traffic flow on the West end of the city. This byway essentially separated the back nine of the golf course into two pieces. Although the traffic congestion improved, drivers using the street were, for the most part, unaware that their vehicles could be the target of stray golf balls hit from the golf course.

It was a wonderful, sunny Saturday afternoon in 2008. I was playing with a fellow from out of town whose name was Faulkner Alexander. He told me that people usually called him "Spud." He apparently was a chubby baby, and his father nicknamed him Spud instead of Potato.

On this particular day, Spud and I were playing quite well and quickly. As I recall, neither one of us had hit a poor shot through 15 holes. As we were walking off the 15th green, I noticed that it had taken us only 2 1/2 hours to play. I mentioned to Spud that we might be able to complete our round in three hours if the pace of play remained the same.

As we approached the 16th tee box I appreciated that the pace of play had stalled considerably. I could see golfers on the tee box, in the middle of the fairway, and on the 16th green. Looking across the course I could see the same situation on the next two holes. It looked like we had encountered a traffic jam and were just going to have to get in line to wait our turn.

Spud and I stopped to wait at the gold, or championship, tee box on the 16th hole while the golfers in front of us hit their shots from the white tee box which was located about 40 yards in front of us. I wasn't paying any attention to the man taking a shot. However, I did hear, "Oh no! Oh crap!"

When I turned quickly to see what was happening, I noticed a golf ball flying to the left of the tee box, over the six-foot chain-link out-of-bounds fence, and striking the windshield of a bright red Dodge pickup with dual wheels coming down the street. At the time, the pickup was the only vehicle I saw on this stretch of road. The vehicle promptly sped up to the entrance of the golf club, made an abrupt U-turn, and sped down the parking lot before coming to stop not far from the 16th tee box. A large, powerfully built middle-aged man hopped out of his pickup and ran toward the tee box. When he arrived by the group of golfers he shouted, "Which one of you bozos hit my truck?"

A bit in awe of this man's behavior, no one said a word.

He then exclaimed, "What are you guys going to do about my broken windshield?"

The burly left-handed golfer who had hit the wayward shot and who was still standing on the tee box with his 1-wood draped over his shoulder replied, "I guess I'll just have to aim farther to right next time."

The incensed driver looked at the group, shouted a few profanities, and stormed back to his pickup. We all watched as the man's vehicle exhaled a large plume of dark smoke before screeching down the parking lot to the exit leaving black skid marks in its wake.

After a few moments the left-handed golfer hit another ball only this time he aimed farther to the right. This ball started out toward the right side of the fairway and made a high sweeping slice across the fairway, past the rough, and settled perhaps a yard from the same out-of-bounds fence.

One of the golfer's companions said, "Ben, you're going to have to start working little bit harder on that slice of yours."

To this the golf replied, "Duh, do ya think?" Then he laughed.

The four golfers got into their golf carts, joked a bit about the incident, and headed down the fairway.

Spud and I thought the incident was pretty funny. With the glacially slow pace of play after this incident, we finally finished our round after three hours 30 minutes. Another day and more lessons learned.

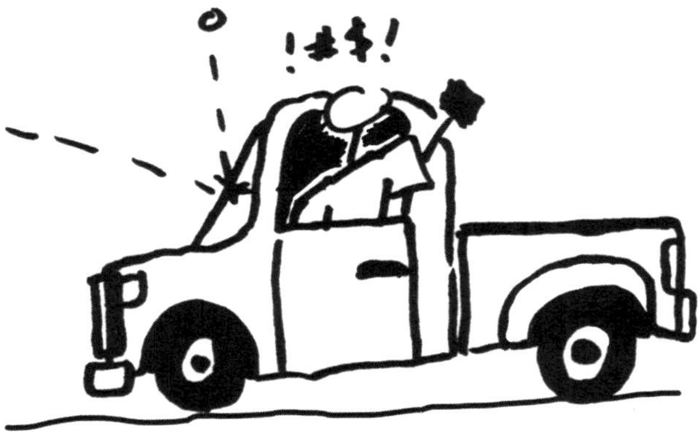

"Don't use the club that worked yesterday. Use a club that will that will get you to the green today."
Anonymous

Sutton's Law

I came upon a threesome on the par 3 third tee box one sunny afternoon in June. The group was waiting for the golfers in front of them to clear the green. They invited me to join them since the pace of play was pretty slow that afternoon. Two of the golfers were walking with their pushcarts and the third golfer was riding in a golf cart.

I thanked them for the offer, introduced myself to each one of the players, and waited for my turn to play. Eldridge was one of the players of the threesome with whom I had golfed several times before. He was a vigorous, healthy appearing man of about 65 years who, as I remembered, played well.

After we had finished the hole, our group started to make our way toward the next tee box. Eldridge was moving slower than I recalled from our previous meeting. I mentioned to Eldridge that he seemed to be walking slower than the last time we played together.

He said, "Doc, I'm just feeling a little bit puny today."

Somewhat in jest, I mentioned to him that with the slow play of golf that day, nobody was going to care if we walked slowly. So all I had to do was to keep up with Eldridge.

The next hole was a par-five 500-yard hole. After Eldridge hit his second shot from the fairway, I noticed that he leaned on his golf club and took some big breaths.

I asked him, "Eldridge, Are you sure you're all right?"

He returned, "All of a sudden I get really tired Doc. I'll just rest here a bit while you take your shot, then I think I'll be okay."

All of a sudden I went into my doctor mode. I had seen people like this before who denied a substantial problem while it was occurring. I told him I thought he should ride in the golf cart.

Eldridge said, “No, that's okay.” After thinking a few moments, however, he said, “Come to think of it that might be a good idea. I'll think I’ll take you up on that offer.”

I called out across the fairway and motioned to the other player who was riding as a single player in a golf cart. I told him that Eldridge was not feeling well, and I thought he should be riding in a golf cart.

Without hesitation, the other player put Eldridge’s golf clubs on the cart and made sure that his playing partner was settled in for the ride. After resting just a short time in the golf cart, Eldridge felt well enough to hit his third shot onto the green. He then two putted for a par.

At the next tee box, which was a par 3 hole, we had to wait once more for the group in front of us to leave the green. In the meantime, being the nosy old family doc that I still am, I started to ask Eldridge questions. He had not eaten anything unusual. He had suffered no vomiting or diarrhea. His appetite was good. As far as he knew, he hadn’t had any fevers or chills. Eldridge said he was walking 18 holes on the golf course just fine up to three days before. He had been mowing his grass at home without any difficulty. By now it was time for all of us to tee off, and since Eldridge was feeling better, our team pressed on with Eldridge continuing to ride in the golf cart.

On the next tee box I asked Eldridge if he had any chest or abdominal pains. He said, “No.”

We played the next hole without incident.

On the tee box of the 7th hole, Eldridge confided to me quietly that he had had a heart attack about 10 years before, and the doctors had placed a stent into one of his heart vessels.

I asked Eldridge if he had regular visits with his heart doctor.

He told me that he had seen his heart doctor about four years before and was told that everything "was good." He was supposed to come back every year, but somehow the time just raced by. Since he felt pretty good, Eldridge allowed the appointments to be missed.

In medical school we learned about Sutton's Law:

A famous unsubstantiated story is that Willie Sutton, the famous bank robber, was asked by a reporter named Mitch Ohnstad why he robbed banks. According to the reporter, he replied, "**Because that's where the money is.**" The quote evolved into **Sutton's Law** which is often invoked to medical students as a metaphor for seeking out the most likely diagnosis when caring for patients, rather than wasting time and money investigating every conceivable possibility.

With this new medical history from Eldridge, my decades of experience in medicine told me that this man had a new heart problem. Even though he was having no chest pain, which occurs only about 20% of the time with people having acute heart attacks anyway, I had strong suspicions he was having atypical angina. I suggested to Eldridge that he see his heart doctor as soon as he could, that meant TODAY!

He told me that he appreciated my concern and that he would call his doctor as soon as he finished the golf round. He then went to the tee box and hit his drive onto the middle of the fairway. Riding in the golf cart allowed Eldridge considerable relief, and he finished the remainder of the round without incident.

As we were leaving the clubhouse I reminded Eldridge to call his doctor as soon as he got home. I insisted that he take an aspirin just in case.

Eldridge promised me he would.

Over the next several months, I did not see Eldridge. Additionally, I noticed that he had not been signing up for senior league golf games on Mondays. Then one warm, sunny Saturday afternoon in mid-August I went to the golf course for some pitching and putting practice. When I saw Eldridge on the putting green, I went over to talk with him and asked, "Hey Eldridge, long time no see. Where have you been?"

Eldridge replied, "Hey Doc, howya doing?"

I told him that I was well as far as I knew. I wondered how he was doing.

He then asked, "Hey Doc, do you remember the last time we played golf and you told me to call my heart doctor that day?"

I told him that I recalled that incident well. I remembered that he was tired, we got him to ride in a golf cart to play, and then he felt better.

He said, "Doc, you've got a darn good memory. I still have trouble remembering where I parked my car in the parking lot this morning." Eldridge then went on to tell me that he had indeed called his heart doctor when he got home. It just so happened that he saw his usual doctor's new young partner that afternoon. According to Eldridge, the young cardiologist looked at his medical record, asked a few questions, performed a heart tracing test, listened to his chest, and, since he was feeling so good at that time, sent him home to take one baby aspirin a day.

I commented something like, "It sounds like you were doing pretty well by then."

Eldridge continued to relate his story. He said the following morning about 10 o'clock he received a call from his usual cardiologist. Eldridge emphasized, "Not his receptionist, but the doctor himself. The cardiologist made a personal call to me." He said the doctor told him to come to his clinic right now.

Eldridge said he asked the doctor what seemed to be the problem. According to Eldridge, the doctor apparently said, "I want you in my office within the hour."

Eldridge apologized to me for taking up so much of my time, and to make his long story very brief, said his cardiologist saw him that morning, he performed an angiogram which revealed that he had two arteries to his heart that were 99% closed, and, before the doctor would let him leave the hospital, Eldridge had an operation to bypass two heart arteries.

As he was recovering from his heart surgery, Eldridge said he asked his cardiologist what he knew that his young doctor friend did not know.

He said his cardiologist told him, "Sutton's Law. Most of the time, to make the right diagnosis we doctors learn to go to where the money is, where the most likely cause is. In your case Eldridge, your heart was the most likely culprit because of your history. And it was."

One of the nearly closed arteries that was reopened is called "The Widow Maker" because if it becomes 100% blocked, the patient dies. Eldridge said the cardiologist told him that he was a lucky man.

On this day, Eldridge was back to playing golf. His heart surgeon said he could start playing golf by putting, AND ONLY PUTTING.

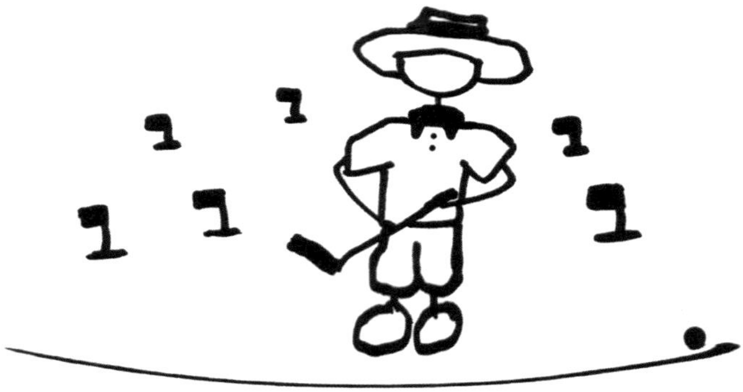

The Good Shot

The game for the day was 2-net-best-balls. After I had signed in about 7:30 in the morning and paid my playing fee of $4, I made my way to the practice area. As I was warming up one of the senior league organizers came up to me and said, “Jim, I know you usually walk the course. But today would you do me a favor and ride along with Hersh.”

I asked if there was a particular reason.

He told me that he just wanted to have someone look after Hersh when he played. Hersh apparently had some significant medical issues and, since I was a physician, the coordinator thought I would be the best one of our foursome to ride along with him.

I agreed. My warm-up this morning was taking my golf cart back to my truck, storing it, and then walking back to the practice area. This may not seem like much, but it was my custom to park my vehicle in the club parking lot at the farthest point from the clubhouse. I always figured that with so many seniors older than me I was able-bodied enough to walk the extra distance.

As I approached the clubhouse a golfer drove up beside me in a golf cart and asked me if I was Jim. When I told him that my name was Jim, he said, “I was told to look for a tall guy with a large brimmed hat. You were the only one that fit that description.”

I chuckled.

The golfer told me his name was Hersh and that he guessed we were playing together that morning.

I confirmed that we were playing on the same foursome, and I understood that we would be starting on hole number 7.

After Hersh confirmed our initial hole assignment, I went into the clubhouse to get a scorecard. Even though the event coordinators gave each foursome an official scorecard for the day's event, I always kept my own score just to validate scores at the end of the round in case our team's official scorekeeper needed to double check every player's scores.

When I got back into the golf cart on the passenger side I could see that Hersh did not look well. He was thin, pale, and spoke slowly. I asked if he wanted me to drive the cart.

Hersh said holding onto the steering wheel kept his hands steady, so he would rather drive if I didn't mind.

I knew that getting into a crash with the golf cart on a wide-open fairway would be most unlikely. While pointing my right arm toward the 7th tee box, I told him, "Let's be off like a herd of turtles!"

On the way to the tee box, Hersh told me that he had Parkinson's disease, and he wanted to play golf as long as he was able. He was 65 years old, which was only three years older than me at the time. By his appearance, I would have guessed that Hersh was closer to 80 years old.

When we arrived at the tee box, Hersh asked me to go ahead and hit because it would take him a little bit of time to get out of the cart.

I told Hersh that we were not in that big of a hurry. We could wait for him to tee off first. Actually, my selfish medical motive for saying this was that I wanted to watch and evaluate a man with an advanced stage of Parkinson's disease.

Hersh agreed to be the first to tee off.

I helped Hersh extract himself from the golf cart. His joints were extremely rigid. His movements were quite slow, jerky, and deliberate. As soon as Hersh released the steering wheel on the golf cart, both of his hands displayed the classic tremor of Parkinson's disease. Hersh then picked out his golf club and a ball. Holding his left arm for stability, I assisted him to the tee box.

Hersh requested that I stand behind him because he told us that sometimes he fell over after swinging his golf club.

I assumed my position behind his back. The other members of the foursome were also prepared to help Hersh if he became unstable.

Hersh asked me to help him tee up his golf ball which I did. Then, assuming a wide-based stance, Hersh hit his ball straight down the fairway perhaps 100 yards. Amazingly, I noticed that his hand tremors went away as he was swinging his golf club. All of us congratulated him on a nice tee shot. Hersh stepped away, braced himself on his golf club so he wouldn't fall over, and waited for the rest of us to make our shots. I then held my partner's arm as he struggled with his rigid gait to make it back to the golf cart.

Sitting in the driver seat, Hersh looked at me, winked, and pronounced, "Now we're off like a herd of turtles!" He laughed.

Before he got out for his second shot, Hersh asked me, "Jim, do you know the definition of a good golf shot?"

I had to admit that I did not.

He replied, "You hit the ball. The ball goes forward, you can find it, and it's not wet! It's as simple as that."

I looked down at Hersh's drive of 100 yards in the middle of the fairway and said something like, "Now that's a quality golf shot."

Hersh replied, "Jim, now you've got it. You've got to make things simple in golf and in life. Now on to our next shot."

I then helped Hersh extract himself from the golf cart, made sure he was steady, and watched this courageous man with a disabling disease hit his second golf shot. My eyes started to have tears just watching him struggle to play the game he loved.

Hersh and I repeated this process for every one of his shots for the next nine holes. Our team did not earn any of the cherished pro shop credits for the day.

However, I learned the real definition of a good golf shot from a real-life pro who knew what he was talking about:

"You hit the ball. The ball goes forward, you can find it, and it's not wet! It's as simple as that."

"Golf is the closest game to the game we call life.
You get bad breaks from good shots; you get good
breaks from bad shots–but you have
to play the ball where it lies."
Bobby Jones

Bibliography

1. The Original Rules of Golf, Professional Golfers Career College, https://golfcollege.edu/original-13-rules-golf/

2. Golf Quotations, Brainy Quote, https://www.brainyquote.com

3. Golf : Naked, The Bare Essentials Revealed, Greg Rowley, 2008

4. www.Wikipedia.com